**Pocket**

# Sports Injuries
## Second Edition

### Mitchell Brooks MD PA

Orthopaedic Surgeon
Plano
Texas


### Roger Evans FRCP

Consultant in Emergency Medicine
Cardiff Royal Infirmary
Newport Road
Cardiff, UK


### John Fairclough FRCS

Orthopaedic Surgeon
Cardiff Royal Infirmary
Newport Road
Cardiff, UK

**Gower Medical Publishing ● London ● New York**

**British Library Cataloguing-in-Publication Data:**

Brooks, Mitchell
Pocket picture guide to sports injuries. – 2nd ed.
I. Title   II. Evans, Roger   III. Fairclough, John
617.1

**Library of Congress Cataloging-in-Publication Data:**

Available on application


**ISBN 1-56375-512-2**

**Project Manager:** Saba Zafar

**Designer:** Pete Wilder
John W Codling
Patrizia Cavalliere
Tim Friers

**Illustrators:** Balvir Koura
Marion Tasker
Mark Willey

**Production:** Susan Bishop

**Publisher:** Fiona Foley

Text set in Sabon and Frutiger by Tradespools, Frome
Produced by Mandarin Offset
Printed in Hong Kong 1992

**Distributed in Southeast Asia, Hong Kong, and Taiwan by:**
APAC Publishers Services
30 Jalan Bahasa
Singapore 1129

**Distributed in Japan by:**
Nankodo Co Ltd
42–6 Hongo 3-chome
Bunkyo-ku
Tokyo 113
Japan

**Distributed in the USA and Canada by:**
J.B. Lippincott Company
East Washington Square
Philadelphia, PA 19105
USA

**Distributed in the UK and Continental Europe by:**
Gower Medical Publishing
Middlesex House
34–42 Cleveland Street
London W1P 5FB
UK

**Distributed in South America by:**
Harper Collins Publishers Latin America
701 Bricknell Avenue
Suite 750
Miami
Florida 3313
USA

**Distributed in Australia and New Zealand by:**
Harper Education (Australia) Pty Ltd
P.O. Box 226
Artarmon
NSW 2064
Australia

## PREFACE

If asked the definition of Sports Medicine 20 years ago, the reply might have been 'orthopaedics for people under 25'. Today, the response is only somewhat true. While Sports Medicine is surely a discipline of Orthopaedic Surgery, it is only partially so.

Over recent years, there have been dramatic changes in the world of sport and consequently in the practice of Sports Medicine. One of the most far-reaching changes has been the internationalization of sports to a degree that was undreamt of only a short time ago. As a consequence of this, we have seen an explosion in the number of participants in sports that are new to countries such as the USA and the UK. With this has come the explosion of information and injury. Accordingly, serious questions about our bodies have evolved, one of which is, how can we prevent injury, and what is the best way to recover? Slowly but surely, medicine has responded. Medical fields such as nutrition, physical therapy, exercise physiology, and biomechanics have become repositories of new and exciting information; they have become subspecialities in their own right and form half the body of the entity that we today call Sports Medicine. The development of the lightweight arthroscope has become the means by which Orthopaedic Surgery has formed the other half of Sports Medicine, and this advance has resulted in the repair of injuries being less time consuming and costly.

Hand in hand with the utilization of arthroscopy has been the increased knowledge of how to treat an injury conservatively, a better definition of what specific injuries are, and which injuries are particularly germane to which athletic activity. As a result, the athletic trainer has become an integral player in the field of Sports Medicine and the first line of defence in the prevention and treatment of most sports injuries at the scholastic level of athletic competition.

So what is Sports Medicine? It is a collection of many healthcare professionals from many disciplines, all trying to achieve the same goal: to keep the public active in the safest possible manner, free from injury, so that they may enjoy their recreational activities.

In view of the changes in Sports Medicine, we have tried to make this book as wide ranging as possible and to illustrate common problems that occur in a variety of sports. While it is not feasible to be completely comprehensive in such a small book, we hope that those doctors, physiotherapists, trainers, and athletes who read it, will find it a useful addition to their sporting libraries.

Many people have helped in the preparation of this book, but special thanks are due to Janet Braddon, Keith Bellamy, Arnold Williams, Professors Ronnie Marks and John Corsellis, Dr CJ Bruton, Saba Zafar, Ken Evans, and Sybil Rees.

**MB**      **RE**
**Texas**   **JF**
            **Cardiff**

# CONTENTS

# THE HEAD AND FACE

Injuries to the head and face commonly occur in contact sports as a result of, for example, a clash of heads. They may be secondary to falls in sports, such as horse-riding, or deliberately inflicted, as in boxing.

Some sports, for example, ice hockey, equestrian sports or cycling, recognize that participation carries a significant risk of head injury, thus the use of protective headwear is either strongly encouraged or made mandatory.

The proliferation of cycling as a recreation has meant an increase in the demand for helmets, and indeed, the purchase of a first bicycle should always be accompanied by that of a first helmet. The public are increasingly aware of the importance of preventing head injuries in sporting and recreational activities. This is especially true where children are concerned, particularly in organized hard-contact sports such as football, ice hockey or interscholastic wrestling.

The explosion of technology in the 80s has assisted in the design and production of effective protective headgear. Lightweight material and high-impact resistant substances have made head- and eyegear more adaptable to specific sports. The utilization of self-inflating liners and advanced suspension systems in football helmets has allowed a further dampening of potentially concussive blows, and this greatly contributes to a reduction of head injuries on the gridiron.

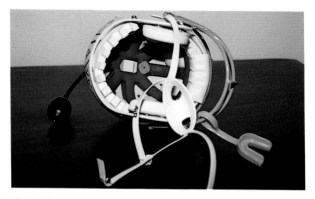

**Fig.1** The suspension system of this football helmet and its self-inflating liner allow a dampening of potentially concussive blows. The yellow gumshield is also illustrated.

Significant blows to the head commonly result in concussive damage to the brain. Frequently, the athlete will experience a transitory episode of disorientation or even a short period of unconsciousness and can be confused on recovery. There may be pre- and/or post-traumatic amnesia. These individuals need to be removed from the playing field and be properly observed and assessed. Consideration must always be given to overnight hospital admission for observation, investigation (skull X-ray, CT scan, and so on) and a.m. reassessment. It is important to remember that the classical presentation of an extradural haemorrhage is that of a lucid interval following the regaining of consciousness. This is followed by a subsequent deterioration of the conscious level as blood accumulates in the extradural space, necessitating urgent surgical treatment.

Head injuries should always be approached with caution, free from any pressures applied by team coaches.

## Soft tissue injuries

The most common soft tissue injuries that occur are contusions and lacerations to the face and scalp, although these may occasionally be complicated by injuries to the underlying bones.

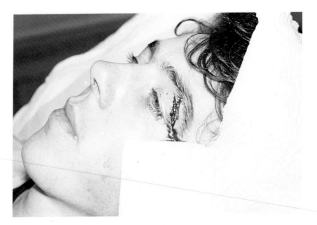

**Fig.2** Laceration to the upper eyelid of a young soccer player.

Lacerations, such as that illustrated in Fig.2, need to be carefully sutured since it is important that the wound edges are accurately approximated to minimize scarring. Cosmetic closure of wounds is not possible in the touchline situation, although this may be attempted due to the pressure which is put on the medical officer to return the player to the field of play as soon as possible. The price of this action is usually a cosmetically unacceptable scar, particularly when wounds are present around the mouth and eyes. Cosmetic closure should be carried out in layers in a controlled situation, using fine suture materials. The use of large, silk sutures in facial wounds with no subcuticular stitches, is not appropriate.

The most serious soft tissue injuries to the facial region are those inflicted on the eye, since temporary, or even permanent blindness, may result. The eye is particularly at risk in sports, such as squash, where the ball is small enough to actually strike the globe itself. The bony margins of the orbit prevent larger balls, for example, those used in tennis or cricket, from doing this.

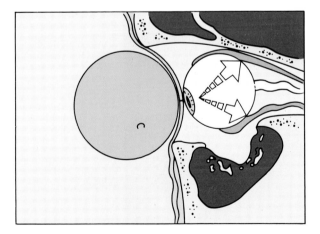

**Fig.3** Diagrammatic representation of a squash ball striking a normal adult eye. The force of impact on the globe, which is considerable, is transmitted in all directions, inflicting damage upon the back of the eye, for example, choroidal rupture or retinal detachment, or even on the bony floor of the orbit causing a 'blowout' fracture.

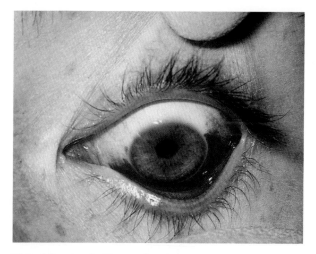

**Fig.4** Subconjunctival haemorrhage in an 18-year-old rugby player caused by a finger accidently being poked into his eye. This type of injury usually settles satisfactorily over the course of 2–3 weeks, provided that there has been no serious underlying damage to the sclera.

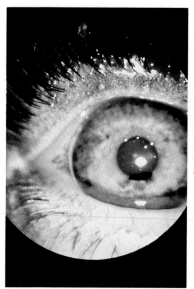

**Fig.5** Corneal abrasion in a 22-year-old rugby player, again caused by a finger. The abrasion stands out well having been stained with fluorescein. Although this is a very painful injury, it is one which usually settles satisfactorily with rest and locally instilled antibiotics.

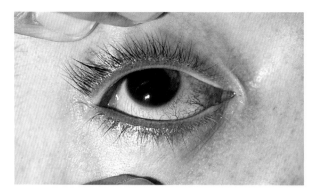

**Fig.6** Hyphema — bleeding into the anterior chamber. This is a more serious, but fortunately less common, eye injury. It is an injury which should not be treated lightly even if the primary haemorrhage is small, since secondary haemorrhage can subsequently occur. This may result in an acute increase in intra-ocular pressure, which occasionally will need to be relieved surgically. It is therefore important to admit patients with such an injury for bedrest and observation until one can be reasonably sure that secondary haemorrhage will not occur. The usual outcome is a complete recovery, as was the case in this 27-year-old ice hockey player who was struck by a puck.

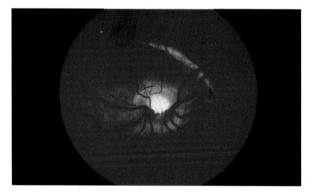

**Fig.7** Injuries to the eyes from squash balls are common. This illustrates the back of the eye of a 26-year-old squash player who has sustained a high-velocity blow from a squash ball. The force of the blow has produced a tear in the choroid, which is typically crescentic and located close to the disc. Management is conservative, and patients usually make a good recovery with preservation of their vision.

Injuries to the eye are preventable in some sports, for example, ice hockey or cricket, by wearing helmets with perspex face masks. Special protective glasses are now available for squash players and are a highly recommended accessory.

Eye injuries also occur in boxing where considerable and recurrent damage is caused to the face. In addition to facial scarring, particularly around the eyes, detachment of the retina may occur. The boxer initially complains of seeing 'floaters', and later, flashes of light. Visual deterioration will eventually become apparent.

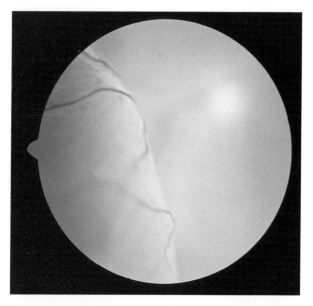

**Fig.8**   Retina, with a rather opalescent appearance, which has 'floated' off the back of the eye. The retina can be clearly seen against the back of the eye, which is out of focus. Urgent ophthalmic referral is required in an attempt to minimize the damage. However, even with early and effective treatment, this is a career-ending condition for a boxer. By courtesy of Baillière Tindall Ltd, from 'Diseases of the eye' by E S Perkins and P Hansell.

A heavy blow to the pinna, an injury which again is most common in the so-called brute sports, can result in a significant amount of bleeding beneath the skin, which is thus stripped off the underlying cartilage. This gives rise to the so-called 'cauliflower ear'.

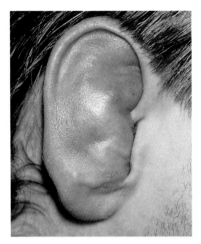

**Fig.9**  26-year-old rugby league player struck heavily on his right ear whilst going down in a scrum. This resulted in a sizable haematoma. Early treatment is necessary if the unsightly, permanent appearance is to be avoided.

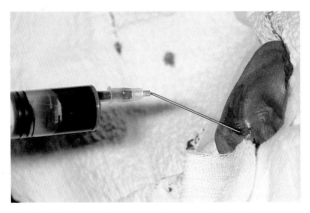

**Fig.10**  Drainage of a haematoma. Treatment of a haematoma should be by immediate drainage using a large bore needle. Subsequently, a firm pressure bandage should be applied to the area to prevent the haematoma reforming.

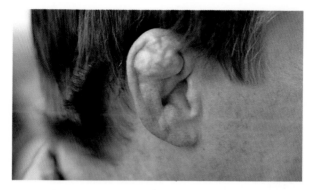

**Fig.11** Chronic 'cauliflower ear' in a retired rugby player whose initial injury was left untreated.

## Infections

Close physical contact, which inevitably occurs in many of the brute sports, results in superficial skin infections being easily passed from one contestant to another. Such infections commonly occur on the skin of the face and can be caused by several different types of organisms. These infections are transmitted because of the abrasion of the superficial layers of the skin, which occurs for instance, in a rugby scrum, or in wrestling.

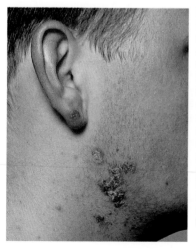

**Fig.12** Superficial skin infection with the herpes simplex virus which occurred in a 22-year-old wrestler. Such lesions can be treated with a topical antiviral agent if they are small and are caught at an early stage. The condition shown is known as herpes gladiatorum or 'scrum pox' and since it is highly infectious, participation in the sport is a contra-indication until healing has occurred.

Occasionally, infections may be bacterial (impetigo or erysipelas) and can also be caused by fungi, such as *tinea barbae*.

## Bony injuries
The nose is the most commonly injured bone in the face due to its prominent position.

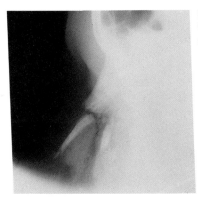

**Fig.13** Lateral view of the nose of a 25-year-old soccer player who sustained this injury as a result of a clash of heads.

If the bones are significantly displaced and/or the airway obstructed, manipulation under anaesthetic is required to correct the cosmetic deformity and clear the airway. In some instances, surgical treatment is delayed until the sportsman has ended his career since these injuries are particularly common in contact sports and it is not unusual for a nose to be fractured several times over the years.

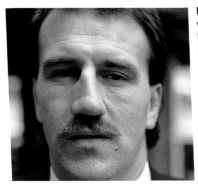

**Fig.14** Rugby player whose nose has been broken four times. He is now aged 34 and corrective surgery will be undertaken when he retires.

The other bones of the facial skeleton, particularly those of the cheeks, are light and prominent and are also commonly fractured in contact sports.

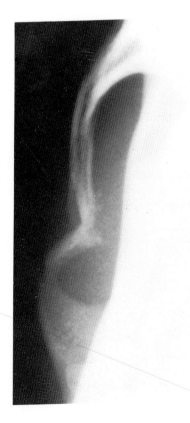

**Fig.15** Sky-line view of the zygomatic arch in a lacrosse player who was inadvertently struck in the face with a stick. A depressed fracture, which was easily detectable, clinically, can be seen, although severe swelling of the soft tissues of the face can sometimes obscure such an injury.

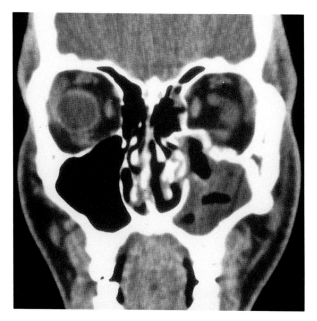

**Fig.16** CT scan of an ice hockey player illustrating a 'blowout' fracture to the floor of the left orbit. Such injuries sometimes result in an ophthalmoplegia due to entrapment of one of the extra-ocular muscles.

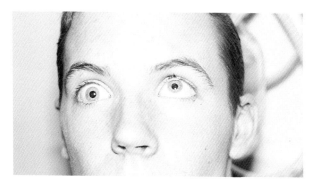

**Fig.17** Ophthalmoplegia. The athlete is being asked to look upwards, which he is unable to do with his right eye. This type of injury requires surgical repair of the orbit and release of the trapped muscles.

The mandible is much stronger than the nasal and cheek bones and usually requires a significant, and sometimes illegal blow, to fracture it.

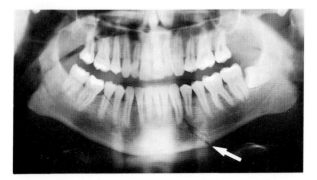

**Fig.18** Orthopantomogram of a 26-year-old soccer player who was struck in the face. There is a fracture through the mandible on his left.

Blows to the face often result in dental injuries, the repair of which can tax the skill of the dental conservator.

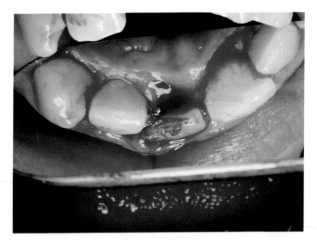

**Fig.19** Intra-oral damage caused by a blow to the mouth with a lacrosse stick.

A sensible piece of equipment for anyone engaged in contact sports is a mouthguard/gumshield.

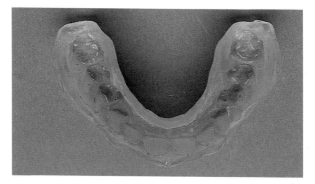

**Fig.20** Mouthguard. The best protection is secured from a guard which is custom-made from an impression of the athlete's teeth.

### Intracranial injury

The vault of the skull is rarely fractured, and unless the fracture is depressed, such injuries are seldom a problem provided there is no underlying brain damage, since linear fractures generally heal satisfactorily. Depressed fractures can be easily missed on plain skull films, thus the investigation of choice is CT.

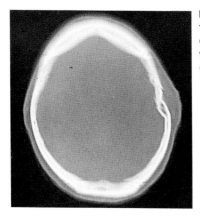

**Fig.21** Depressed fracture of the left side of the skull in a golfer who had been struck by a club.

Any significant blow to the head inevitably causes some damage to the brain and, recurrent injures, even if relatively minor, can have a cumulative effect. Boxers, particularly those of past generations who fought many hundreds of bouts, sustain frequent injuries of this nature, which can result in a chronic, progressive post-traumatic encephalopathy, the so-called 'punch-drunk' syndrome.

The appearance of a cavum in the septum pellucidum is an early sign of damage consequent upon recurrent intracranial injury. In life, this is now best demonstrated by CT or MRI.

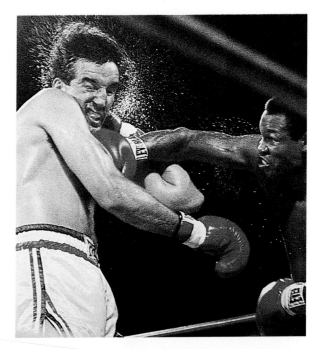

**Fig.22**  World Heavyweight Championship fight between Gerry Cooney and Larry Holmes. Cooney has just been in receipt of a punch to the side of his face which has caused the head to spin violently, throwing off a spray of perspiration. The brain has thus been exposed to both torsional and concussive forces, which inevitably result in neuronal damage.

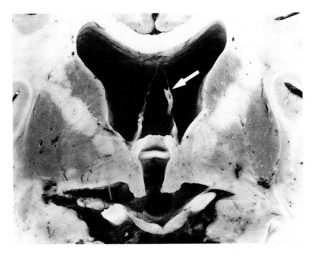

**Fig.23** Coronal section through the anterior horns of the lateral ventricles of a 63-year-old ex-boxer. A cavum septum pellucidum can be seen, with only a few strands of septum having survived. This man was found derelict and infested shortly before his death. Several neurological abnormalities which were related to his brain damage were detectable on examination.

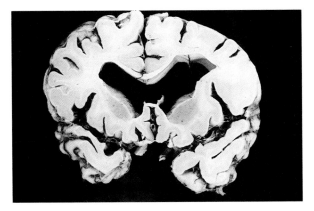

**Fig.24** Coronal section through the brain of a 77-year-old ex-boxer. The boxer had fought over 700 bouts and by the age of 50 was staggering and dysarthric. He died demented and doubly incontinent in a psychiatric facility. Note the dilated ventricles. A ventricular diverticulum can also be seen.

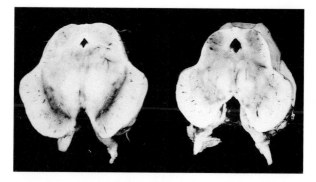

**Fig.25** Two transverse cuts through the mid-brain of, on the right, a 69-year-old ex-boxer who was 'punch-drunk', and on the left, an age-matched control. Note the pigmentation of the normal substantia nigra is quite obvious whilst that in the boxer is barely noticeable. Damage to this area is thought to account for the Parkinsonian features of the 'punch-drunk' syndrome.

A subdural haematoma is a more acute neurological problem associated with boxing, which can occasionally be fatal. Such an extracerebral bleed can also occur following injuries in other sports, such as horse-riding.

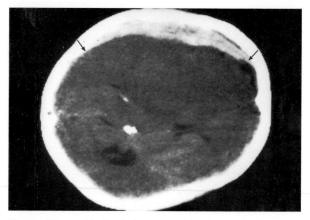

**Fig.26** CT scan of the head of a 20-year-old ice hockey player who sustained a heavy blow during a practice session when he was not wearing protective headwear. The extradural haematoma that has resulted lies between the two black arrows.

# THE NECK

Injuries to the neck vary from minor, soft tissue strains of ligaments and muscles, to catastrophic damage to the spinal cord following fractures and fracture/dislocations.

## Soft tissue injuries

Acute torticollis is a painful condition which can occur in athletes following sudden, violent movements of the head and neck. Severe pain which starts in the evening or on the day following the event is usually experienced in the muscles of one side of the neck. The head and neck are held fixed, often at an angle, and the pain is exacerbated by movement.

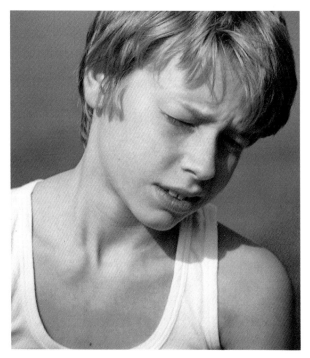

**Fig.27**  Ten-year-old gymnast who landed badly following a vault, and later in the day presented with pain and marked muscle spasm in the trapezius and sternomastoid. Treatment is with rest, heat, administration of local nonsteroidal anti-inflammatory drugs (NSAIDs) and physiotherapy.

Occasionally, an injury sustained during a sporting activity is the result of deliberate foul play. Contact sports, by their nature, offer enough violent physical involvement, and anyone caught deliberately inflicting an injury upon a fellow player should be severely dealt with.

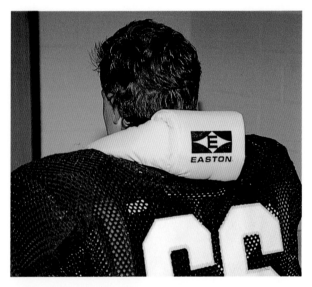

**Fig.28** The use of a neck roll in football can decrease the incidence of hyperextension injuries. In addition, a 'horseshoe' can minimize stinger or burner injuries since it limits the extent of lateralizing forces on the neck.

### Bony injuries

The cervical spine is constructed so as to allow great flexibility, the head being able to move freely over a wide range. The cost of this freedom of movement is that the cervical spine is less stable than other areas of the spine. In the neck, the facet joints are relatively narrow and flat, allowing free movement, and as a consequence of this, they are prone to degenerative change and at risk of dislocation. The main support for the structure is provided by the broad interspinous ligament and the anterior and posterior longitudinal ligaments.

In addition, the spinal canal itself in the cervical region is quite narrow relative to the size of the spinal cord. Thus, if further narrowing occurs due to a dislocation or a disc prolapse, or secondary to a degenerative process with osteophytes, the cord is easily impinged upon. This causes symptoms and sometimes permanent damage. Indeed, a congenital narrowing of the canal or an extradural defect must be sought out in the high-school level football player who continuously sustains 'stinger/burner' injuries (traumatic brachial plexalgias).

There can be no sadder sight in sport than that of a young athlete who is tetraplegic following an injury to the cervical spine. Bony injuries to the neck occur in gymnastics, equestrian sports, football, rugby and the high-risk sports such as racing in all-terrain vehicles and hang-gliding.

When a neck injury has occurred on the field of play and neurological damage appears to have been inflicted, it is absolutely vital that the medical/paramedical personnel who take the athlete to hospital do not exacerbate the damage. The athlete must be removed carefully, preferably by trained people, using the appropriate rescue apparatus. The use of a correctly sized hard collar such as the Philadelphia collar is an ideal method for temporarily stabilizing the injured neck. The collar is a flat sculptured piece of stiff plastic which can

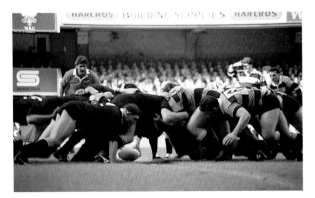

**Fig.29**  The rugby scrum is one area of the game where a risk of injury exists, since the pressures placed upon the necks of the participants are enormous. Those who play in the front row are in most danger, particularly when an untoward event occurs, such as a sudden scrum collapse.

easily be passed behind the patient and then assembled. Patients with spinal injuries should be supported and transported on a firm, inflexible stretcher or frame, of which several types are available. A useful type is the scoop stretcher which is made of lightweight aluminium and which can be disassembled to allow for adjustments, enabling it to fit the individual patient. Separate halves are then slipped beneath the patient and locked into place, and the patient is lifted and transported to hospital.

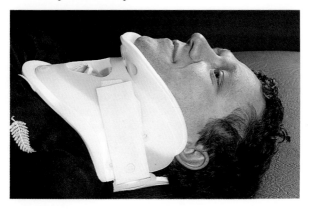

**Fig.30** Philadelphia-type collar assembled to support and immobilize the neck.

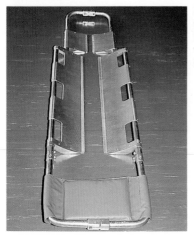

**Fig.31** Assembled scoop stretcher which is infinitely adjustable within a normal range of heights.

If no collar is available, the head and neck must be kept supported and immobile, with light traction applied to the neck in a longitudinal direction. Movements of the head and neck must be kept to a minimum.

In order to place the patient onto the stretcher, he should be 'log rolled' with the head, trunk, pelvis and limbs being turned as a single unit, while the cervical spine is stabilized by the medical officer who applies gentle traction.

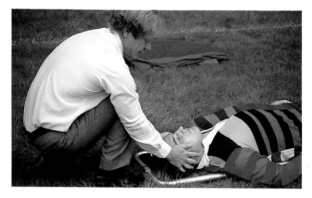

**Fig.32** In the absence of a support for the neck, the head is being supported on the stretcher by a medical officer who is maintaining light, manual traction in a longitudinal direction.

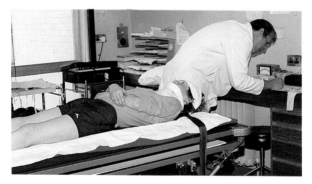

**Fig.33** Neck supported in a stiff collar. The patient was taken to hospital for appropriate clinical and radiological assessment. In addition to plain X-rays, CT and MRI are now important investigative tools in the management of spinal injuries.

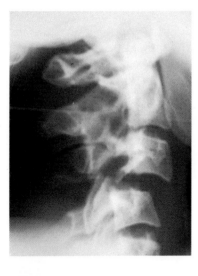

**Fig.34** Lateral X-ray of the neck of a 36-year-old horse-rider, who fell, landed awkwardly and sustained a C3/C4 unifacet dislocation. She was neurologically intact and underwent reduction of the dislocation. Local fusion and wiring of the C3/C4 interspinous area was also carried out.

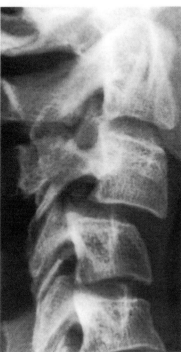

**Fig.35** Bifacet dislocation at the C3/C4 level in a 28-year-old rugby player who was injured in a scrum collapse. Unfortunately, this resulted in complete tetraplegia, the almost inevitable consequence of such an injury.

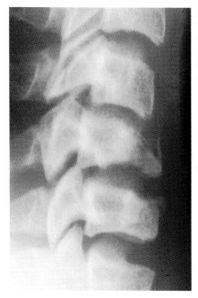

**Fig.36** Lateral view of the neck of a 21-year-old man who dived into shallow water, striking his head on the bottom and suffering a hyperflexion injury to his neck. A 'teardrop' fracture of the anterior part of the body of C5, together with a crush fracture of the body of C6, has occurred.

The inevitable result of long-term stress, with increased neck loading, is the premature onset of degenerative change. This can occur in young men, producing symptoms of aching pain in the neck often associated with paraesthesia in the hands, and pain over specific nerve root distributions.

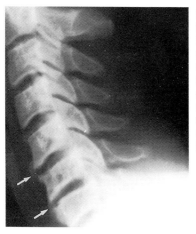

**Fig.37** Lateral view of the cervical spine of a 28-year-old football player showing degenerative changes with loss of disc space and the presence of anterior osteophytes most particularly at the C5/6 and C6/7 levels (arrowed).

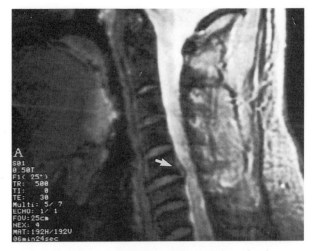

**Fig.38** MRI of the neck of a 34-year-old football player showing a disc protrusion at the C5/6 level (arrowed). He presented following an injury late in the game which left him with pain and weakness in his right arm.

## THE SHOULDER AND UPPER ARM

The shoulder is a free-moving joint with a large range of polyaxial movement. As a consequence of this, it is relatively unstable. Injuries to the shoulder and upper arm can either be traumatic or may result from overuse. Dislocations, subluxations and fractures account for a majority of the former, while overutilization of a tendon, joint capsule, ligament or muscle, resulting in painful function, defines the latter.

These overuse syndromes are caused by the repetitive movements necessary to compete successfully in sports such as swimming, rowing and baseball. Alternatively, they may be secondary to the immense strains placed upon the joints in gymnastics and weightlifting. Athletes whose activities involve the use of the shoulder tend to overdevelop the muscles around the joint: an example of this is the wheelchair athlete who undertakes long-distance races in his or her chair. The shoulders, under these conditions, are subjected to tremendous strains and, furthermore, to overdevelopment. Wear and tear in the area is severe.

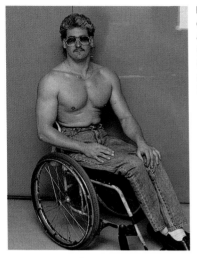

**Fig.39** Highly competitive wheelchair athlete. Note the massive upper body development compared with the atrophic, paralyzed lower limbs.

If the muscles of the upper limb are subjected to sudden, severe strains, for example, in weightlifting, javelin throwing or baseball pitching, muscle tears, ruptures and tendon avulsions can occur.

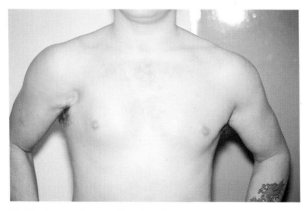

**Fig.40** Ruptured pectoralis major which occurred in this young weightlifter while he was snatching 90kg. Unfortunately, he was unable to return to competitive weightlifting, although after some months he resumed work as a labourer.

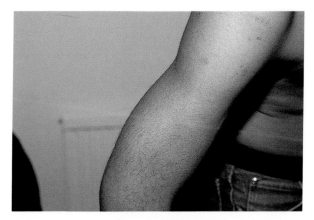

**Fig.41** Rupture of the triceps which occurred in a 27-year-old boxer while he was involved in a work-out using the heavy bag. As with the athlete described in Fig.40, this man was unable to return to boxing at his previous level despite a prolonged period of rehabilitation.

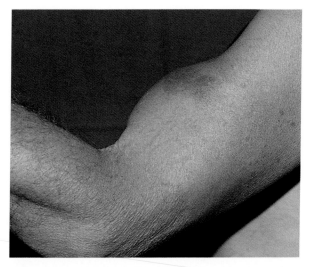

**Fig.42** Ruptured long head of biceps in a 47-year-old cricketer who had previously undergone a repair for recurrent dislocation of the shoulder. In general, the long head tends to rupture in degenerative conditions rather than secondary to overuse, and it is only an occasional problem in younger people.

Although repair is sometimes possible for muscle/tendon injuries of the type described in Figs.40 and 42, the results in high-class athletes are generally not good and few are able to return to competition at their former level.

Aching pain in the shoulder, with restriction of movement and limitation of function, is particularly common in athletes whose sport involves repetitive overhead use of the arm, such as tennis, baseball and swimming. The problem is known as the impingement syndrome and is due to bony and soft tissue structures around the shoulder impinging one upon the other: for example, the head of the humerus on the corocoacromial arch. This causes inflammation in adjacent tissues (bursa and rotator cuff). While not strictly an overuse syndrome, impingement is one of the most common causes of shoulder pain in an athlete, and if recognized and treated early, is usually reversible. It may be detected by the impingement test.

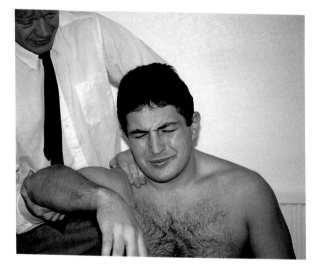

**Fig.43** Forceful elevation of the arm while stabilizing the scapula, compresses the irritated tissues under the corocoacromial arch and reproduces the athlete's pain.

In mild cases, restriction of activity for several weeks is often sufficient to alleviate the problem, together with the use of locally applied NSAIDs. A local injection of a steroid may be required later, and if the injury is more severe, it is occasionally necessary to resort to surgery.

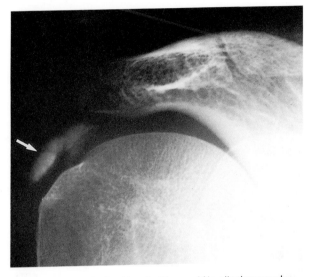

**Fig.44** AP X-ray of a shoulder of a 31-year-old javelin thrower who had a minor aching pain in the joint, which increased in severity over the season, eventually stopping him from competing. Calcification (arrowed) in the supraspinatus tendon, a condition that is often linked with other degenerative conditions in the rotator cuff, can be seen. The problem was relieved by administration of a local steroid injection, although it was several months before the patient returned to competitive sport.

## Bony injuries

The bone which is most likely to fracture in the shoulder girdle is the clavicle; this fracture is usually caused by falls onto the point of the shoulder.

In cases where the falls are upon the point of the shoulder, where the clavicle does not break, damage to the ligaments around the acromioclavicular joint often occurs, with consequent subluxation. The patient is exquisitely tender directly over the acromioclavicular joint, and shoulder movements are grossly limited. Treatment is as for a fractured clavicle.

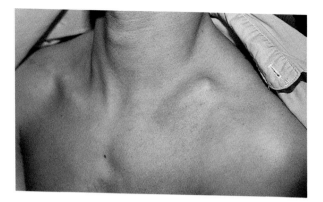

**Fig.45** Characteristic appearance of a midshaft fracture of the clavicle in a young hockey player who slipped whilst playing on an artificial pitch. The fracture is obviously displaced but, any attempt to try to reduce this displacement by conservative methods is destined to be unsuccessful, for example, with figure of eight bandages which are difficult to apply, and which always loosen. Rest for 3–4 weeks in a broad arm sling is all that is required, followed by a course of physiotherapy to enable the athlete to regain a full range of movement.

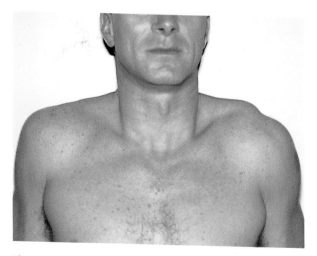

**Fig.46** Twenty-eight-year-old football player who has sustained a subluxation of his left clavicle.

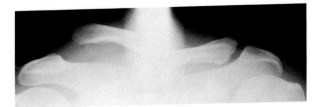

**Fig.47** X-ray of both shoulders of a 25-year-old rider who fell onto her right side. The subluxation of the acromioclavicular joint is obvious; however, this appearance has been accentuated by first, comparing it with the normal left side and secondly, by making this a weight-bearing view in which the individual is holding a heavy weight in her right hand, thus exaggerating the separation between the clavicle and the acromial process.

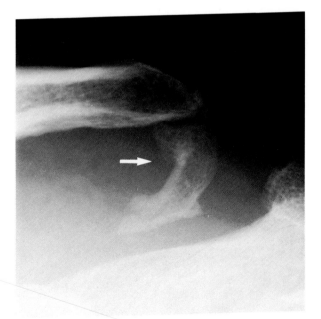

**Fig.48** AP X-ray of the left shoulder of a 29-year-old footballer, who has chronic acromioclavicular subluxation. There is obvious ossification in the ligament beneath the lateral end of the clavicle.

Recurrent or severe injuries to the shoulder can result in damage to, and subsequent calcification/ossification of, the ligaments running between the clavicle, coracoid and acromion. The abnormality is often picked up as an incidental finding on X-ray and generally speaking it does not affect the functioning of the joint.

The shoulder is the most commonly dislocated large joint, particularly in contact sports and secondary to falls, for example, from horses.

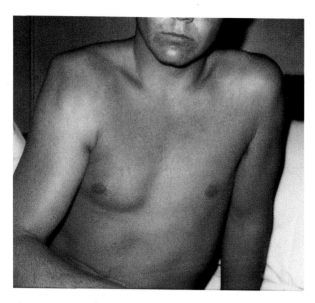

**Fig.49** 21-year-old rugby player who fell onto his right shoulder. Loss of the normal contour of the shoulder can be seen. Movement in the joint was very restricted although the acute pain had settled by the time the player arrived at hospital. Treatment of this condition is by reduction under adequate analgesia/anaesthesia but it is important to confirm the diagnosis by taking an X-ray. This will exclude any associated bony injury, since occasionally an upper humeral fracture may mimic an anterior dislocation.

Anterior dislocations are by far the most common type and are generally obvious on clinical examination; radiographic confirmation is also straightforward. Posterior dislocations are notoriously deceptive on an AP X-ray, and an axial view is imperative to confirm the diagnosis.

Another unusual type of dislocation is the subglenoid dislocation or luxatio erecta, where the head of the humerus is forced downwards into the subglenoid region and the arm lies raised above the head.

If the dislocation has severely damaged the capsule of the joint, there is always the possibility of the injury recurring when sporting activity is resumed. Under these circumstances, surgical stabilization is frequently undertaken.

Shoulder pads can be worn in some sports in order to protect joints that are weakened by previous injuries.

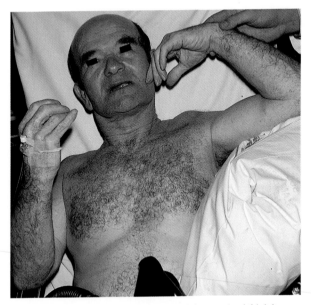

**Fig.50** Subglenoid dislocation in a man who sustained this injury whilst diving off a 5m board.

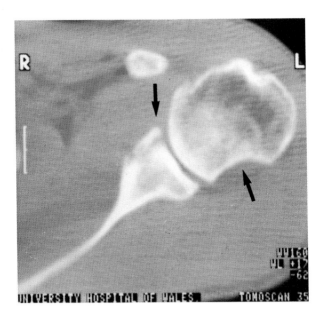

**Fig.51** Two lesions are characteristically produced by recurrent dislocation, these being the Hill-Sachs lesion (hatchet defect) on the posterior surface of the humeral head, and the Bankart lesion, which is a result of damage to the inferior cartilaginous rim of the glenoid. These abnormalities are illustrated in this CT scan of the shoulder of a 28-year-old soccer player.

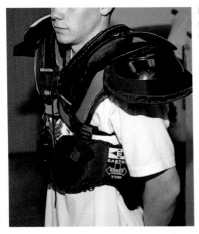

**Fig.52** Protective shoulder harness as worn by a football player. He is also wearing a rib-pad extension which helps prevent injuries, particularly in quarterbacks.

## THE LUMBAR SPINE

Sports, which stress the lumbar spine in particular, include rowing, weightlifting and gymnastics. Certain aspects of other sports, for example, fast bowling in cricket and propping in rugby football, are also major causes of back problems amongst athletes.

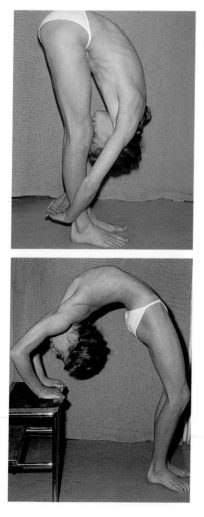

**Fig. 53** Thirteen-year-old gymnast who is demonstrating the range through which her spine can easily move.

As gymnastics becomes more competitive and children begin this sport at an earlier age, care must be taken that damage is not caused to the immature skeleton by over-enthusiasm for training and competition.

In the adolescent male athlete with back pain, it is important to exclude Scheuermann's disease, which is a type of osteochondritis affecting the vertebral ring epiphysis.

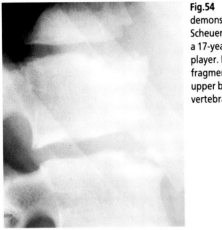

**Fig.54** X-ray demonstrating Scheuermann's disease in a 17-year-old squash player. Note the fragmentation of the upper border of the vertebral body.

In general, Scheuermann's disease is usually found in the thoracic spine and may give rise to a round-back deformity if the vertebrae become wedged. The complaint mainly affects adolescent boys and should be managed conservatively.

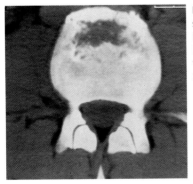

**Fig.55** CT scan of the spine of a 19-year-old hockey player showing a large defect in the vertebral body due to Scheuermann's disease.

Fractures of the lumbar spine are rarely seen secondary to direct trauma other than in the high-risk/high-velocity sports. Stress fractures of the pars interarticularis, however, are not unusual in sports where the spine is subjected to severe, repetitive strains.

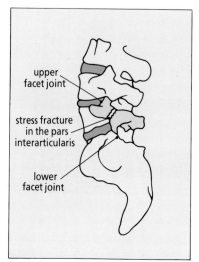

**Fig.56** Diagrammatic representation of a stress fracture of the pars interarticularis. The pars is the area of bone running between the superior and inferior facet joints of the vertebrae. The fracture line running across the pars is the spondylolysis.

upper facet joint

stress fracture in the pars interarticularis

lower facet joint

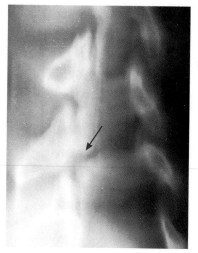

**Fig.57** Tomogram of the lumbar spine of a 27-year-old softball pitcher, illustrating a spondylolysis at the L4/5 level (arrowed).

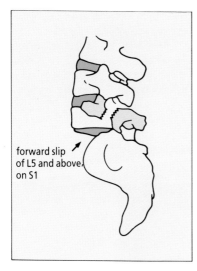

**Fig.58** If the stress fractures are bilateral, the upper and lower parts of the spinal column are no longer connected by bone, and the superior part of the spine can start to slip forward on the inferior part, causing a spondylolisthesis, as shown.

forward slip of L5 and above on S1

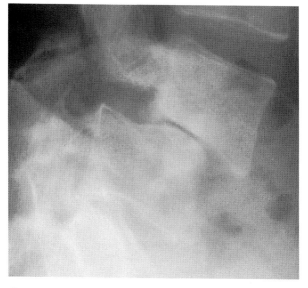

**Fig.59** Lateral view of the lumbosacral spine in a 20-year-old gymnast with spondylolisthesis at the L4/5 level. The risk of slippage is most marked in the younger athlete.

Occasionally, athletes present with back pain and sciatica, and under these circumstances, neurological examination is mandatory since a prolapsed disc may be impinging on the nerve roots. The most common level for a disc prolapse is at L5/S1 and in these circumstances the ankle jerk is often impaired. The MRI scan is the investigation of choice at present.

There is no doubt that participation in certain sports to a high level, such as gymnastics, brings with it the penalty of early degenerative changes in the spine.

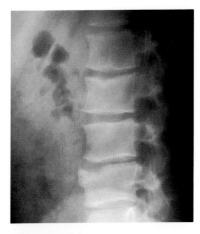

**Fig.60** Lateral X-ray view of the lumbar spine of a 28-year-old gymnast. Note the multiple endplate abnormalities with an anterior interosseous nuclear herniation at the L3/4 level, resulting in a limbus vertebra. There is disc-space narrowing at the L4/5 level.

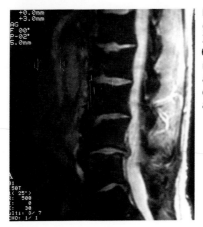

**Fig.61** MRI of the gymnast whose plain X-ray is illustrated in Fig. 60. All the discs in this region are abnormal, and there are central disc bulges at the L4/5 and L5/S1 level.

# THE ELBOW AND FOREARM

The elbow allows flexion and extension at the humero-ulnar joint, and pronation and supination at the radio-ulnar and radiohumeral joints.

In the sportsman, the joint is stressed by all throwing activities, which are severely restricted if the elbow cannot fully extend. In racquet sports, the elbow becomes the fulcrum of movement and the forces placed upon it are considerable.

## Soft tissue injuries

Any activity that involves the hand being used for gripping, will cause contraction of the forearm muscles, particularly those arising from the common extensor origin of the lateral epicondyle. The musculature arising from the medial epicondyle (common flexor origin) is utilized to a lesser extent and is thus not as frequently problematic. Persistent forceful repetitive strains on the sites of insertion, particularly on the lateral aspect, may produce inflammatory changes causing

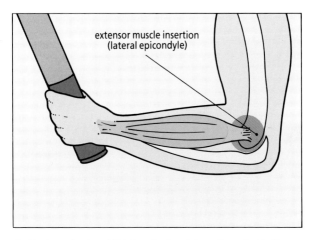

**Fig.62** Lateral epicondylitis (tennis elbow). Stress is applied to the relatively small area over the lateral side of the elbow, where the extensor muscles originate. Repeated stress on this region can produce inflammation, and an overuse type of epicondylitis may result.

pain at the elbow. The most common example of these over-use syndromes is tennis elbow.

Lateral epicondylitis is common in any sport where repetitive forceful wrist extension occurs. In tennis, this condition is commonly caused by an improper grip, hitting behind the ball on the backhand, a racquet with a head that is too small, or by stringing under excessive tension. A similar chronic inflammatory condition known as 'golfer's elbow' occurs on the medial epicondyle, and this also may be caused by faulty technique or by using clubs that are inappropriately sized.

Treatment is by modification of technique and training, use of simple analgesics or NSAIDs, and physical therapy to develop the forearm musculature. Avoidance of the offending activity for 3–6 weeks is absolutely essential. In recalcitrant cases, local steroid injections may be useful, and with failure of these modalities, surgical release of the area may be necessary.

## Bony injuries

When children participate in sports that involve vigorous throwing actions, they are susceptible to recurrent injury around the elbow joint. This is most commonly seen in little league pitchers, producing the condition known as 'Little League elbow', and X-rays of the area reveal fragmentation in the region of the epiphyses. Treatment is with rest and reduction and/or modification of the sporting activities for several months. In severe cases, it may not be possible to continue with the sport.

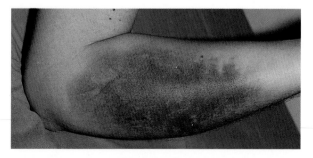

**Fig.63** Right forearm of a 22-year-old exponent of knockdown karate who blocked a kick with the limb during a contest. Fortunately, there was no evidence of any underlying bony damage.

The most common fracture to the elbow region is one involving the radial head/neck. However, an injury which is rather more serious and a well-recognized problem, particularly in gymnastics, is the supracondylar fracture.

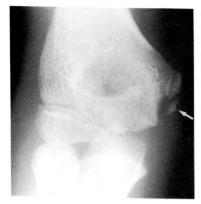

**Fig.64** AP view of the elbow of an 11-year-old baseball pitcher. Note the fragmentation around the medial epiphysis (arrowed). This is the so-called Little League elbow.

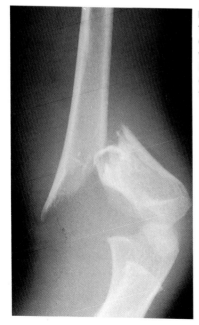

**Fig.65** Lateral view of the elbow of a 10-year-old gymnast injured whilst trampolining. Note the grossly displaced supracondylar fracture.

Clinically, the deformity in cases such as that described in Fig.65, can be confused with a posterior dislocation of the joint, hence it is essential to take X-rays rather than attempt an immediate reduction of a suspected 'dislocation'. Furthermore, when the displacement is as marked as this, there is a danger of damage occurring to the nerves and blood vessels of the antecubital fossa. Although this type of fracture normally heals well after reduction and immobilization, there is frequently a reduced range of movement at the elbow (particularly extension) which makes participation in some sports difficult.

Another serious fracture which occurs at the elbow is that to the olecranon since it disrupts the extensor apparatus. Such fractures can occur secondary to a fall onto the flexed elbow, or are sometimes caused by a sudden, violent contraction of the triceps which avulses its insertion. In young adults, it is essential to reattach this fragment in order to regain full joint function.

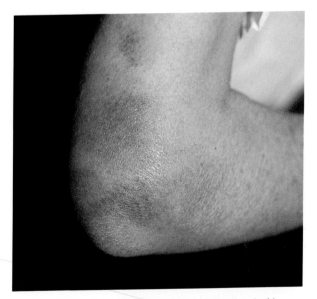

**Fig.66**  Bruising around the extensor aspect of the elbow in this tennis player has been produced by the bleeding which has occurred secondary to a fracture of the olecranon.

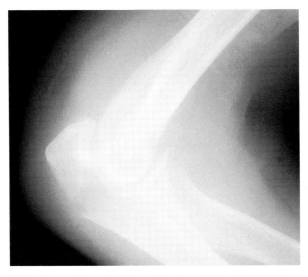

**Fig.67** Lateral view of the X-ray of the elbow illustrated in Fig.66. The fractured olecranon is clearly demonstrated.

Dislocations of the elbow are seen in gymnastics and some contact sports. The dislocation is normally a posterior one and is occasionally associated with a fracture of the proximal ulna or radius.

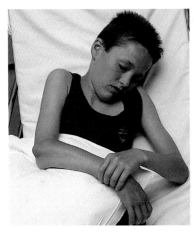

**Fig.68** A young gymnast in obvious pain, secondary to a dislocation of the right elbow.

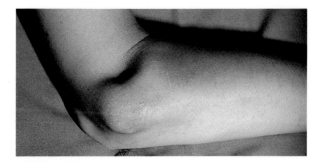

**Fig.69**   Close-up of the characteristic appearance of a dislocation of the elbow. Reduction should only be undertaken under adequate anaesthesia/analgesia. Recovery is normally complete, although extension of the elbow may take some time to return to normal.

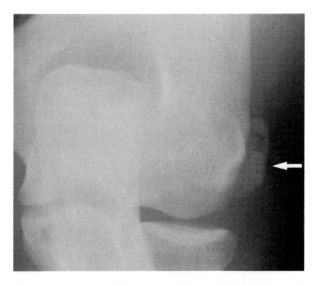

**Fig.70**   Heterotopic calcification around the joint is a complication of a dislocation of the elbow and indeed of other elbow injuries. It is demonstrated in this view of the elbow of a 26-year-old rugby player who dislocated the elbow whilst making a tackle with his arm extended. Note the small, calcified mass adjacent to the lateral epicondyle which has developed in the two months following the dislocation. The concern often expressed about this uncommon condition is misplaced, since, unless it is severe, it is normally asymptomatic.

Occasionally, athletes will present with limitation of elbow movement, sometimes associated with locking of the joint, and with pain and swelling. This is often due to osteochondritis, which generally involves the capitellum (Panner's disease), with the resultant extrusion of a loose body into the joint cavity.

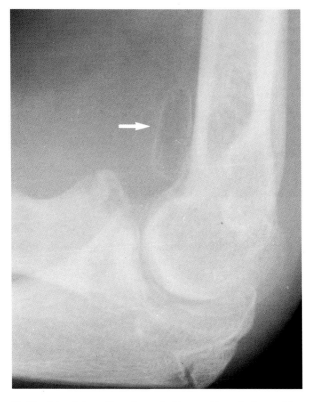

**Fig.71** Lateral view of the elbow of a 13-year-old tennis player with a large loose body (arrowed) in the joint. This was secondary to an osteochondritis of the radial head and was later removed at operation.

Repetitive stress and the associated minor trauma to the joint, which occurs in certain sports, will result in degenerative (osteo-arthritic) changes developing in the elbow. In normal circumstances, the elbow is not commonly affected by this condition.

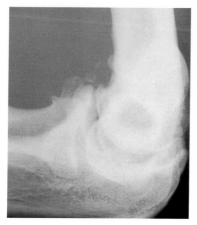

**Fig.72** Lateral view of the elbow of a 41-year-old ex-javelin thrower. Note the extensive degenerative changes, with numerous loose bodies.

Fractures of both the radius and ulna, or a 'night stick' type fracture of one of these bones only, is seen in a variety of sports.

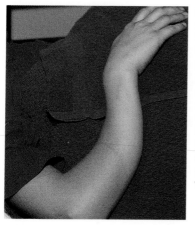

**Fig.73** Fracture of the radius and ulna, which has occurred in a young female gymnast injured whilst trampolining. It is particularly important in such patients to obtain correct anatomical alignment when the fractures are reduced and fixed, otherwise supination and pronation of the forearm will be affected.

# THE WRIST AND HAND

Wrist and hand injuries are an inevitable consequence of certain sports, including those which involve catching or throwing hard balls, for example, cricket or baseball, those where the hand itself is used to strike the ball, for example, in volleyball or handball, or those where the hand is used as a weapon, as in boxing and some martial arts. In addition, the delicate, mechanical function of the hand can become the site of inflammation as a result of overuse.

## Soft tissue injuries

Overuse injuries, such as tenosynovitis, are common where repetitive activity of the wrist/hand is necessary, as in rowing.

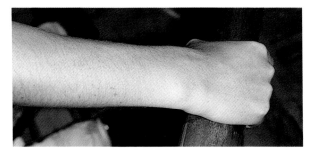

**Fig.74** Grip of a 21-year-old oarswoman. At this stage of the rowing sequence the oar has been pushed away from the body and the wrist is palmar flexed, with the oar being firmly gripped.

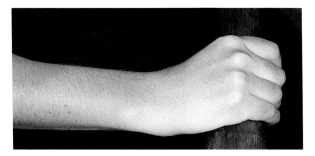

**Fig.75** The oar is being pulled close to the body, and the wrist has been snapped back into dorsiflexion.

These rapid and repetitive wrist movements, undertaken while the oar is being firmly gripped, lead to severe stressing of the extensor tendons and can produce a tenosynovitis which is often difficult to treat.

When sportsmen are catching or striking hard balls on a repetitive basis, minor soft tissue, and occasionally bony, injuries, are inevitable. These injuries are common, and because the damage tends to be cumulative, permanent deformities may result. Under these circumstances, serious functional impairment of the hands can result since it is usual for sportsmen to continue to play despite 'carrying' minor injuries.

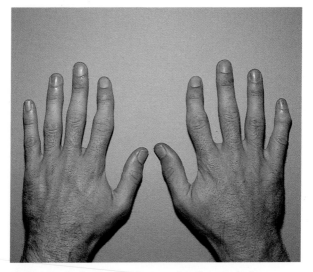

**Fig.76** Hands of a 24-year-old county wicketkeeper who has deformities of the fingers. He already has impaired finger flexion and a reduction of grip strength in the left hand.

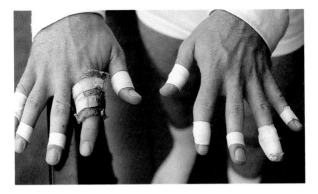

**Fig.77** Protective strapping used by a wicketkeeper prior to taking the field. Light chamois leather inners and heavy leather and rubber gauntlets are placed over this.

In certain sports, such as some martial arts, the hands are used as weapons and also for striking and shattering hard objects for display purposes.

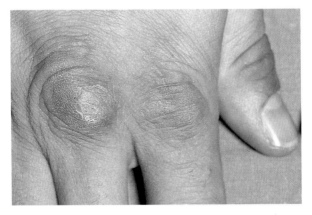

**Fig.78** Right hand of a 24-year-old 'breaker', an exponent of karate who shatters solid objects, such as tiles, bricks and planks. The callouses over the metacarpophalangeal joints are obvious and are the result of continuous practice. Surprisingly, only a few bony injuries occur, although these athletes do present with painful wrists and hands, as do boxers.

Skiing is another common cause of hand problems. The injuries occur particularly around the first metacarpophalangeal joint with damage to the ulnar collateral ligament, the so-called skier's (gamekeeper's) thumb.

In the acute stage of skier's thumb, there is tenderness around the first metacarpophalangeal joint, and an attempt to demonstrate instability is difficult since it is extremely painful to stress the joint. When the acute injury has settled, the unstable joint can be X-rayed and the subluxation clearly shown by stressing.

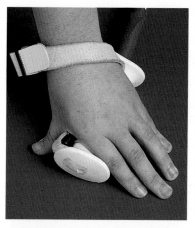

**Fig.79** Ski-pole being driven into the first web space as the result of a fall. This abducts the thumb and causes disruption of the ulnar collateral ligament. This injury is common in both snow- and dry-slope skiing and prevention is difficult. However, some protection may be obtained by wearing gloves where the thumb is syndactylized to the index finger.

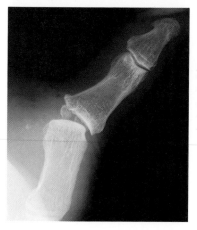

**Fig.80** X-ray appearance of an unstable first metacarpophalangeal joint. Stress applied by the examiner has caused the joint to open up. Good results are possible from surgical repair of this type of lesion.

## Bony injuries

As with many other joints, the wrist has an area which is subject to a type of osteochondritis. In Kienbock's disease, the lunate becomes avascular and fragmented.

As with many of the other osteochondritides, treatment of Kienbock's disease is with rest until it resolves, although various surgical procedures have been attempted in order to speed up the healing process. Unfortunately, in some athletes residual deformity due to osteo-arthritic degeneration may cause persistent carpal pain and stiffness.

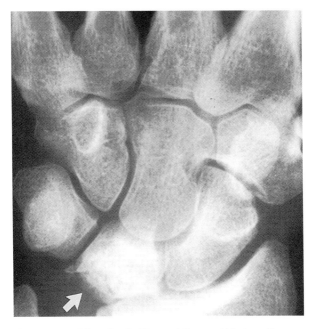

**Fig.81** X-ray of the wrist of a 20-year-old boxer which shows the characteristic appearance of the lunate in Kienbock's disease. The boxer presented with a dull, aching pain in his wrist which had been present for over 18 months.

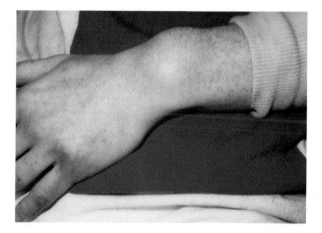

**Fig.82**   Wrist of a 15-year-old rugby player who has a swelling over the dorsum of the joint secondary to an underlying Salter-Harris type II fracture of the distal radius. Fortunately, this healed normally and there was no impairment of function.

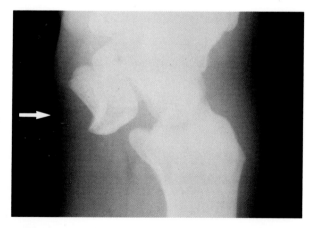

**Fig.83**   Lateral X-ray of the wrist of a 25-year-old weightlifter who, following a clean-and-jerk manoeuvre, suddenly felt pain in his wrist and tingling in his fingers, and consequently dropped the bar. The X-ray shows a dislocated lunate; this is commonly overlooked. The dislocation was readily reduced under general anaesthetic, and the paraesthesia which was related to median nerve compression, resolved in the month or so following the injury.

Falls onto the outstretched hand are common in many sports, and result in either bony, or soft tissue, damage. The treatment for these types of injuries is no different in the sportsman or the nonsportsman. Unfortunately, however, a residual disability due to such injuries may prevent some athletes from continuing in their sports.

The scaphoid is another carpal bone which is frequently damaged in a fall onto the outstretched hand and again is an injury which can be missed on X-ray, with catastrophic results for the athlete (avascular necrosis of the bone and subsequent osteo-arthritic degeneration of the wrist joint).

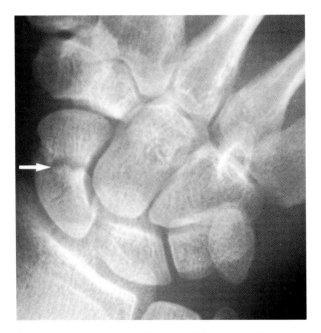

**Fig.84** Fracture of the waist of the scaphoid in a 22-year-old soccer player. On his first visit to hospital, only AP and lateral views of the joint were obtained and the faint fracture line which was apparent across the waist of the bone, was missed. He returned seven days later and on this occasion, special scaphoid views were obtained and the fracture spotted; these magnified views were obtained on screening with the wrist held in ulnar deviation, a manoeuvre which 'opened up' the fracture to make it more visible.

Another fracture of the carpus, which is linked with sporting activity, is that to the hook of the hamate. It is notoriously difficult to demonstrate this fracture on plain X-ray and if it is suspected, the investigations of choice are triple-phase technetium 99 bone scanning and CT scanning. The injury is usually the result of the handle of a baseball bat, tennis racquet, golf club, cricket bat, or hockey or ice hockey stick forcibly striking the palmar aspect of the user's wrist.

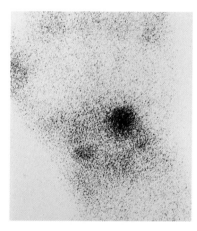

**Fig.85** Technetium 99 bone scan of the wrist of a 30-year-old baseball player who presented with pain after receiving a blow on the flexor aspect of his wrist from the handle of his bat. There is an area of increased isotope uptake over the hamate, and subsequent CT scanning revealed a fracture to the hook of this bone.

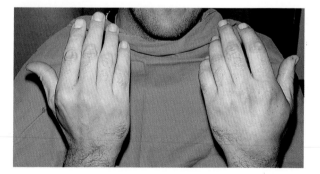

**Fig.86** Hands of a goalkeeper demonstrating swelling of the left hand due to fractures of the second and third metacarpals. These injuries kept him out of league action for six weeks.

Fractures and dislocations of phalanges and fractures of metacarpals are an occupational hazard of those who play in certain positions in sports such as baseball (catchers) and soccer (goalkeepers).

The fifth metacarpal is the most likely to fracture, usually at the neck (the boxer's fracture). Often, there is some associated forward displacement of the head of the bone into the palm.

If the patient is asked to extend the fifth finger there is frequently a loss of extension, and although a variety of splinting methods can be applied, it is difficult to stop the fracture falling into a volar displacement. Fortunately, the malunion which occurs has very little functional consequence. Although this is called a boxer's fracture it rarely occurs in the sport itself, either professional or amateur, since gloves are used and the hands are taped. In the majority of cases, it is associated with illicit use of the fist during contact sports!

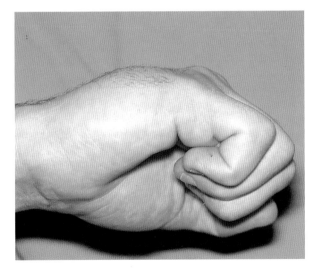

**Fig.87** Fracture of the neck of the fifth metacarpal of the right hand of a 26-year-old defensive linesman. Note the deformity, swelling and loss of the knuckle.

Fractures and fracture/dislocations of the first metacarpal are common sequels of falls while snow skiing. As with skier's thumb, they are caused by the ski-pole acting as a fulcrum in the first web space where the first metacarpal wraps. If the pole straps are also through the first web space, they act as an additional force levering the first metacarpal.

A similar injury is the so-called Bennett fracture/dislocation. In this type of injury, it is important to ensure that reduction is maintained; surgical intervention is occasionally required.

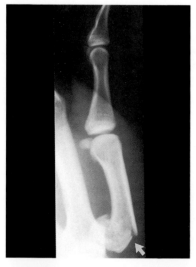

**Fig.88**  Fracture of the base of the first metacarpal (arrowed) sustained by a 28-year-old skier.

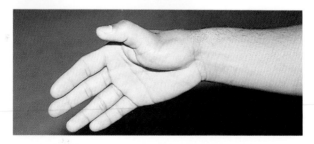

**Fig.89**  Hand of an exponent of full-contact karate who mis-hit an opponent in a bout. The thumb is dislocated at the metacarpophalangeal joint.

Dislocations of the digits, provided they are not open or associated with significantly displaced fragments, can usually be reduced on the field. Dorsal dislocations of the metacarpophalangeal joints may be simple or complex. Simple dislocations usually reduce easily, but complex ones often require surgical reduction. The complex dorsal dislocation can be distinguished by dimpling on the volar aspect of the joint. Its appearance is not as dramatic as its simple counterpart, since the proximal phalanx is usually only hyperextended slightly. On X-ray, the sesamoid is usually seen within the widened joint space. The irreducibility of complex injuries is related to the interposition of soft tissues, usually the volar plate.

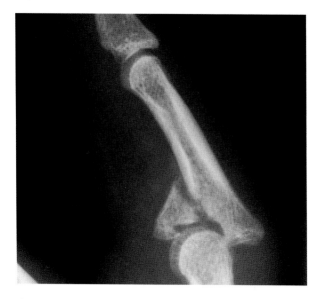

**Fig.90**  Right middle finger of a 28-year-old cricketer who was struck on the finger whilst fielding. The joint immediately became swollen, markedly restricting finger movement. The player did not present for three weeks on the incorrect assumption that this was merely a soft tissue injury. It can be seen that there is a grossly displaced fracture to the base of the middle phalanx which has disrupted the joint. He now has an almost useless finger with an exceedingly restricted range of movement. Although immediate surgery would have been difficult in this situation, reconstitution of the articular surface should have lessened the deformity, improved function and reduced the risk of subsequent osteo-arthritis.

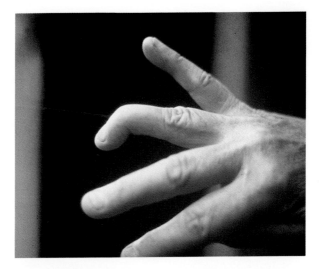

**Fig.91** Characteristic appearance of a 'mallet' finger deformity in a 23-year-old goalkeeper who was struck on the tip of his finger by the ball. This resulted in a sudden, forced hyperflexion at the distal interphalangeal joint which has avulsed the long extensor tendon. The result is an inability to extend the terminal phalanx. This type of injury is generally treated conservatively with rest in a 'mallet' finger splint for six weeks; this holds the distal interphalangeal joint in full extension.

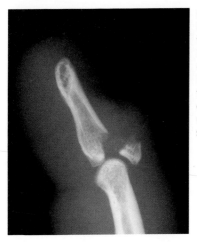

**Fig.92** Fragment of the bone at the base of the terminal phalanx, which has been avulsed by the extensor tendon. In this instance where the fragment was large, operative fixation was undertaken, using a small screw.

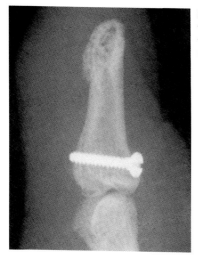

**Fig.93** Operative fixation of the avulsed fragment described in Fig.92, using a screw.

# THE PELVIS AND THIGH

The majority of injuries to the pelvis and thigh usually involve the soft tissues, since a considerable amount of force is required to fracture a femur or disrupt the pelvis. The latter type of injuries are generally only seen in vehicular sports. Common soft tissue problems include strains of the muscles, particularly the adductors, and muscle haematoma, caused by direct blows or intrinsic muscle ruptures.

## Soft tissue problems

### Infections

Fungal infections are common in sportsmen; these may occur as a result of maceration of the tissues of the perineum when the athlete perspires and/or from the skin being rubbed by underclothes and athletic supports.

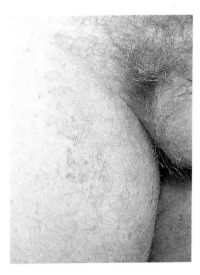

**Fig.94** *Tinea cruris* in a 26-year-old tennis player. Treatment is with use of a topical antifungal, such as econazole, and strict hygiene. Unfortunately, relapse is frequent.

## *Injuries*

In certain contact sports, including soccer and rugby, blows to the hips, pelvis and thigh, usually from the knees and boots of the opponent, or secondary to being struck by the ball, are an occupational hazard.

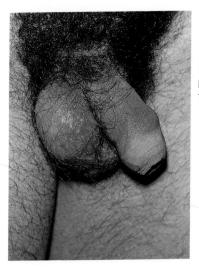

**Fig.95** Severe bruising to genitalia with an underlying, traumatic haematocele. This injury in a 20 year-old soccer player was caused by a fiercely driven soccer ball.

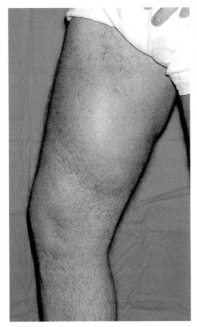

**Fig.96** Large haematoma, the contents of which are obviously fluid. This 36-year-old soccer player was struck on the thigh by the knee of an opponent seven days prior to this photograph being taken.

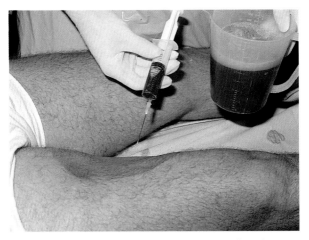

**Fig.97** Haematoma, following aspiration. Over 0.5 l of blood was removed prior to a pressure dressing being applied. If an infection sets in, serious problems can ensue, therefore this procedure has to be performed under strictly sterile conditions.

Frequently, haematomata in the region of the thigh are intramuscular, and if the correct treatment of ice, rest and support is not applied, then occasionally, heterotopic ossification may occur.

In addition to haematomata secondary to blows, muscle tears of varying severity are commonly seen, particularly if explosive starts, or sudden bursts of sprinting are required.

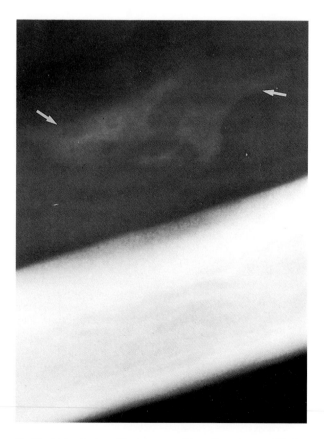

**Fig.98** Heterotopic ossification or myositis ossificans (arrowed) in the thigh of a 29-year-old basketball player who was complaining of recurrent muscle tears. This was treated conservatively with rest and later with the use of a continuous passive movement machine.

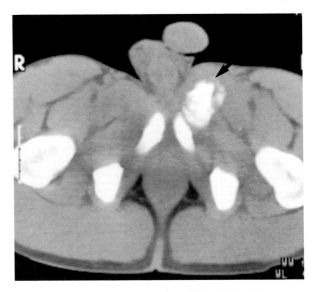

**Fig.99** CT scan demonstrating myositis ossificans in the adductor muscles close to their origin from the pelvis, as a result of a severe tear some three months previously.

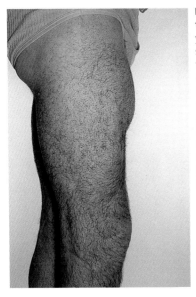

**Fig.100** Lateral view of the right thigh of a 20-year-old sprinter. The sprinter experienced a tearing pain in the front of his right thigh during a training session. A rupture of rectus femoris can be seen. His straight-leg raising was reasonable, and conservative management of the rupture was undertaken.

In many sports, athletes complain of pain around the groin, the ubiquitous 'groin strain'. This is frequently due to chronic problems at the origin of the adductor muscles from the pelvis. Such injuries in the early stages may respond to rest, nonsteroidals (topical and systemic) and physiotherapy.

It is important to ensure that athletes warm up, cool down and undertake stretching exercises before competing, especially if they are heavily muscled, since such people often have tight hamstrings and adductors.

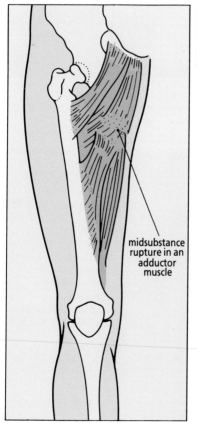

**Fig.101** Adductor strain. The strain can occur in any part of the muscle but is frequently at, or near, the origin.

midsubstance rupture in an adductor muscle

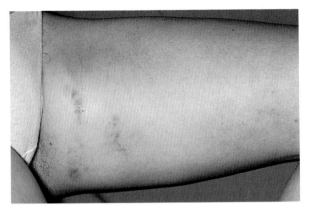

**Fig.102** Bruising seen on the inside of the thigh of a 21-year-old female exponent of karate who had an acute tear of her adductor muscle.

## Bony injuries

Sudden, explosive movements, as in sprinting and long jumping, can occasionally cause problems when muscles avulse part of the pelvis from where they take origin.

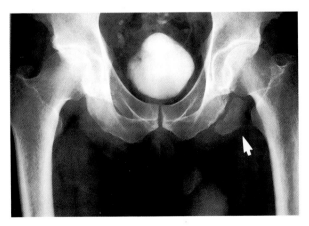

**Fig.103** X-ray of a 25-year-old hurdler who has avulsed part of his ischium from which the hamstrings take origin. This injury occurred in his youth and did not appear to have adversely affected his career.

Another source of pain in the groin is the so-called osteitis pubis, which is a noninfective condition caused by repetitive overstressing of the area. This can result in instability between the two halves of the pelvis.

First-class footballers are particularly at risk of instability, and fusion of the symphysis may sometimes be necessary where instability can be demonstrated on screening.

Whilst fractures of the pelvis due to direct trauma are uncommon, stress fractures of the pelvis and hips do occur, particularly in female long-distance runners.

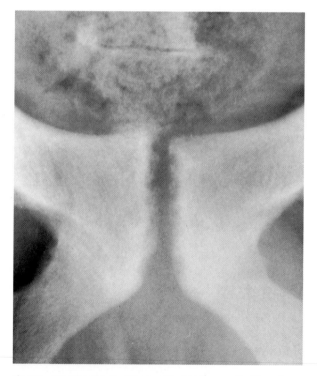

**Fig.104** Osteitis pubis in a 22-year-old wicketkeeper. The X-ray shows that there is irregularity on both sides of the symphysis pubis, and flamingo views confirmed instability.

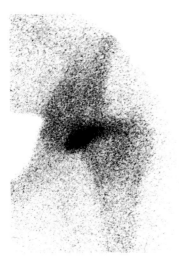

**Fig.105** Stress fracture of the neck of the left femur in a 44-year-old female marathon runner who complained of pain in the hip. Physical examination was normal, apart from the fact that there was some reduction in internal rotation. Plain X-rays were unremarkable. The technetium 99 bone scan shows an area of markedly increased uptake in the region of the femoral neck.

Although there has been some disagreement as to the incidence of osteo-arthritic changes in the hips of athletes in later life, it is now generally accepted that excessive trauma to the joints does lead to early degenerative changes.

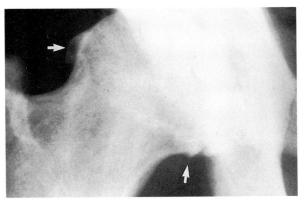

**Fig.106** X-ray of the right hip of a 34-year-old man who was a fanatical roadrunner, covering in excess of 100 miles per week. Degenerative changes, far in advance of what would normally have been expected, can already be noted. As well as narrowing of the joint space and some subchondral sclerosis, there are osteophytes (arrowed) on the femoral head.

## THE KNEE

The knee is particularly at risk in many sports, especially those that involve heavy physical contact, such as soccer, football, basketball and rugby, because of its position in the lower limb and its structure as a simple hinge joint.

Soft tissue injuries to the knee are common in any sports medicine practice and usually involve the collateral or cruciate ligaments, or the menisci.

### Soft tissue injuries

#### *Ligament injuries*
Ligament injuries can occur when a severe stress, either direct or shearing, is applied across the knee.

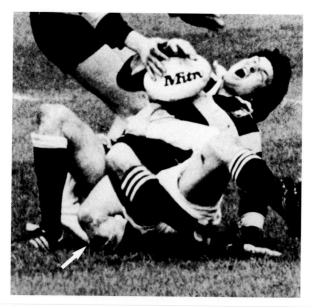

**Fig.107**  A rugby player's left leg is trapped, and with his tackler's leg acting as a fulcrum, the tibia is being forced forward (arrowed). Marked anterior displacement of the tibia upon the femur has occurred and this has produced an anterior cruciate tear, a medial collateral ligament tear, and a torn medial meniscus, the classic triad of O'Donohue.

Swelling is the initial reaction of the knee to an injury and is caused by bleeding into the joint (haemarthrosis), or by an effusion of synovial fluid. It is usually clinically evident (particularly when it is compared with the uninjured side) and it inevitably causes some restriction of knee movement.

If the swelling occurs shortly after the patient has sustained the injury, then it is likely to be due to bleeding into the joint, secondary to severe intra-articular damage, for example, complete rupture of the anterior cruciate.

It is often not possible to establish an accurate diagnosis shortly after an injury, due to the pain and muscle spasms which make clinical examination difficult. However, it is important when inspecting and palpating the knee to look for swelling, bruising and areas of local tenderness over ligaments and joint lines.

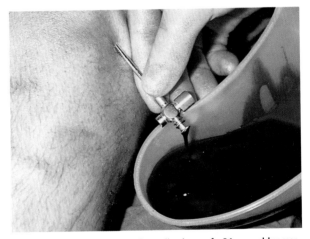

**Fig.108** Drainage of the acutely swollen knee of a 34-year-old soccer player who sustained a twisting injury. This is a useful procedure since it identifies the type of fluid which is causing the swelling and also helps to ease the pain by relieving distension. It is carried out under sterile conditions using gloves and skin disinfectant, for example, povidine iodine in alcohol. In this particular instance, over 100ml of blood was drained from the knee. Subsequent arthroscopy revealed complete midsubstance rupture of the anterior cruciate and it was some 12 months before the player was able to resume his sporting career following the reconstruction and reinforcement of the damaged ligament with a polypropylene graft.

If a patient is seen some weeks after injury, normal routine knee examination, together with an accurate history, can point to a diagnosis in the majority of cases. Plain radiology is usually the first investigation undertaken after noting the patient's history and carrying out as exhaustive an examination as is possible under the circumstances. Many knee injuries only involve the soft tissues, and X-rays appear normal; however, in some cases, minor bony abnormalities indicate significant underlying damage.

An indication of a significant previous injury to the medial collateral ligament is the so-called Pellegrini-Stieda lesion. This lesion represents heterotopic ossification in the ligament secondary to its partial avulsion.

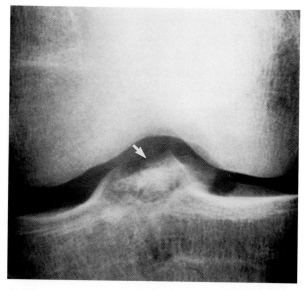

**Fig.109** X-ray of the knee of a 27-year-old squash player showing a tibial spine that has been avulsed by the anterior cruciate. When the incident occurred, the player experienced severe pain in the joint, and also heard a 'pop' from the knee; this is not uncommon in acute anterior cruciate disruption. If not recognized, injuries such as this can lead to severe, chronic instability. In this particular case, the avulsed fragment was replaced using screw fixation.

When the acute phase of a ligament injury has settled, it is possible, without the use of an anaesthetic, to demonstrate rupture of ligaments and instability of joints by taking stress radiographs.

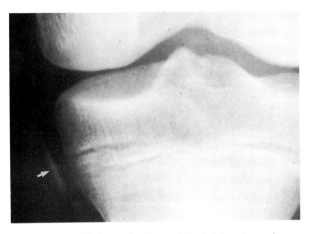

**Fig.110** X-ray of the knee of a 19-year-old badminton player who had injured the joint eight months previously. The medial ligament was still slightly tender on firm palpation, and examination revealed a valgus instability of the joint due to medial collateral ligament damage. The Pellegrini-Stieda lesion is arrowed.

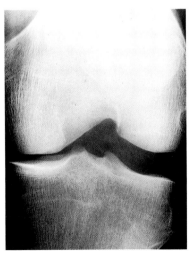

**Fig.111** Stress view of the knee in a 30-year-old hockey player who injured his leg some six months previously. When valgus stress was applied to the knee, the joint 'opened' medially since the medial collateral ligament was ruptured.

## Meniscal injuries

The other intra-articular structures which are frequently damaged are the menisci, most commonly the medial. Diagnosis is based upon a history of pain, swelling, clicking and locking of the joint, together with episodes of the knee 'giving way' unexpectedly. Examination may reveal tenderness over the damaged structure, and occasionally, a definite 'click' may be felt when moving the knee passively through its range.

The advent of MRI has provided a noninvasive method for diagnosing torn menisci and damaged cruciate ligaments. As this technique becomes more available, it will probably be the investigation of choice for knee injuries though the cornerstone of diagnosis remains to be an accurate history and thorough physical examination.

The management of knee injuries has been revolutionized by the introduction of the arthroscope, and whilst other joints, for example, the shoulder or the ankle, can be arthroscoped, most experience has been obtained in examination of the knee. This is because not only is it large but it is accessible and easily manipulated. A cannula is inserted into the superolateral or superomedial aspect of the knee, through which sterile fluid is run into the joint in order to wash blood

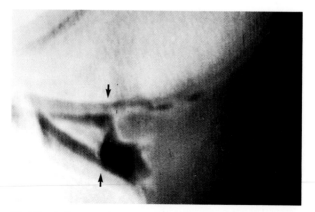

**Fig.112** Arthrogram showing a tear (arrowed) of the posterior horn of the medial meniscus in a 26-year-old cross-country runner.

and minor debris out of the cavity and cause distension. The arthroscope is inserted through a small hole to one side of the patellar tendon, and the intra-articular structures, such as menisci and ligaments, can be inspected through separate portals so that an accurate diagnosis can be made.

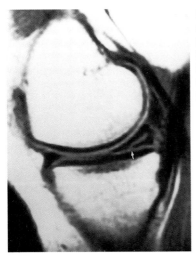

**Fig.113** MRI scan showing a tear in the posterior horn of the medial meniscus (arrowed) in the knee of a 28-year-old baseball player.

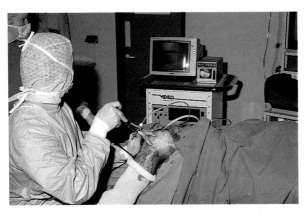

**Fig.114** Arthroscopy being performed on the knee of a 30-year-old table tennis player. The surgeon observes the image of the interior of the knee on a TV screen, the image being produced from a small video camera connected to the arthroscope.

With the development of small, precisely engineered instruments, none of which has a diameter of more than 0.5cm, many intricate diagnostic and therapeutic procedures can now be undertaken during arthroscopy. The aim of the surgeons is to remove as little as possible of the damaged meniscus, as this will help to prevent premature degenerative change in the hyaline cartilage which is known to be hastened by total meniscal removal.

Occasionally, meniscal lesions present with cysts along the joint line usually on the lateral aspect. The athletes usually have a history of a previous knee injury, and the swelling appears gradually over a period of months. The tear in the meniscus appears to act as a flap-type valve and synovial fluid accumulates in the cyst causing a swelling.

Irritative prepatellar bursitis is a type of 'housemaid's knee' which occurs in many sports, such as wrestling and some martial arts; it is a cause of anterior knee pain and swelling. Treatment is with rest, physiotherapy and NSAIDs, although occasionally a steroid injection may be required.

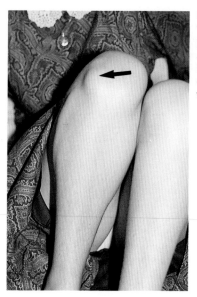

**Fig.115** Lateral cyst of the knee joint in a 32-year-old tennis player. Arthroscopy showed a horizontal cleavage tear of the meniscus which was excised.

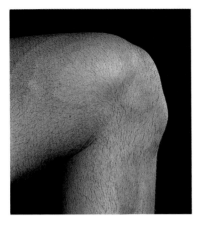

**Fig.116** Prepatellar bursitis in a 23-year-old weightlifter who, after initially failing to respond to rest and conservative management, responded to a local steroid injection.

## Bony injuries

The combination of pain, swelling, locking and giving way in a knee joint may well be due to a lesion of one of the menisci, but occasionally it can be caused by another entirely unrelated condition, osteochondritis dissecans, with an associated intra-articular loose body. This condition is thought to be due to a problem with the vascular supply to an area of bone, and the site most commonly affected in the knee, is the lateral side of the medial femoral condyle. If the fragment is large enough, some surgeons suggest fixation to prevent its separation, or alternatively, the area may be drilled to encourage the formation of fibrocartilage.

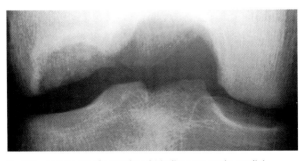

**Fig.117** Large area of osteochondritis dissecans on the medial condyle of a 30-year-old golfer.

Osteochondritis dissecans can occur in bones other than the femur, for example, the patella, and in joints other than the knee, for example, at the ankle, in the dome of the talus.

When an osteochondral fragment becomes detached, it will float freely in the joint space as a loose body. If it becomes trapped between the articular surfaces it will probably interfere with the function of the joint, causing pain and locking.

Osteochondritis involving the patella can sometimes affect the lower pole ossification centre, giving rise to the so-called Sindig-Larsen-Johannson disease, which is similar in appearance on X-ray to Osgood-Schlatter disease.

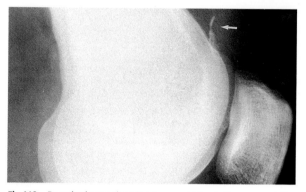

**Fig.118** Detached osteochondral fragment lying in the suprapatellar pouch in the right knee of a 23-year-old basketball player.

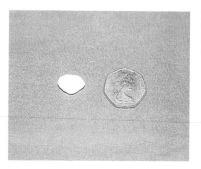

**Fig.119** Loose fragment shown in Fig.118 following its removal with arthroscopy.

Trauma can produce a picture similar to osteochondritis dissecans when for instance, an athlete has a fall onto the point of the flexed knee. This may produce an osteochondral fracture with subsequent separation of the fragment, and permanent damage to the articular surface of the joint.

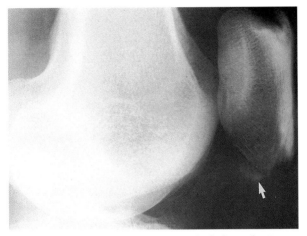

**Fig.120** Sindig-Larsen-Johannson syndrome in the knee of a 19-year-old long jumper. Note the fragmented appearance of the lower pole of the patella.

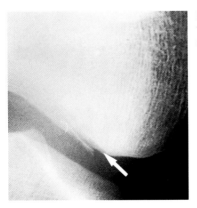

**Fig.121** Osteochondral fracture in a young skater.

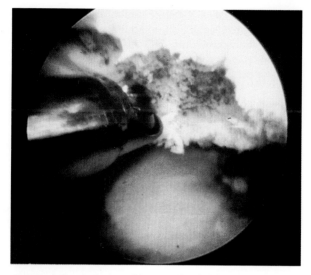

**Fig.122** Arthroscopic view of the osteochondral fracture shown in Fig.121. Detachment of a large piece of hyaline cartilage and some underlying bone, has occurred.

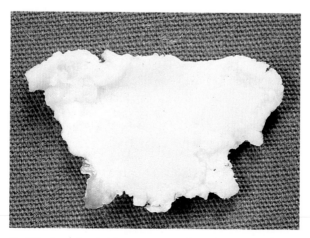

**Fig.123** Osteochondral fragment removed at arthroscopy. Under favourable circumstances, and where the fragment is large, it may be worthwhile to attempt to reattach the piece of bone/cartilage in order to restore the integrity of the articular surface.

Anterior knee pain is a common complaint, and when found in a young, athletically inclined teenager, it is likely to be due to Osgood-Schlatter disease, the pain being sited, in and around, the tibial tubercle. The tubercle is often enlarged and tender, and the pain experienced is worse on exertion. The condition is an apophysitis of the tubercle and is best treated conservatively; most cases settle, although the condition may recur up to the onset of skeletal maturity.

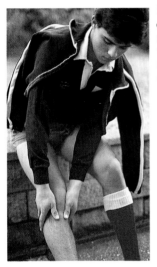

**Fig.124** Fifteen-year-old rugby player with a swollen, tender tibial tubercle in the right knee due to Osgood-Schlatter disease.

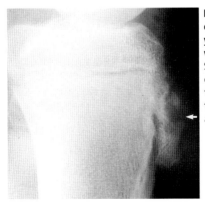

**Fig.125** Radiograph of the right knee of a young baseball player who has Osgood-Schlatter disease. The characteristic fragmentation of the tibial tubercle is arrowed.

Bi- or tri-partite patellae are normal variants of the patella, although occasionally, an inexperienced observer will mistake one for a fracture. Usually they are asymptomatic, but some patients complain of the onset of knee pain during athletic activity, which is probably due to abnormal tracking of the patella.

As with many of the other bones in the lower limb, stress fractures of the patella occur as an overuse injury in several sports.

Recurrent dislocation of the patella is usually found in young people, being more common in girls. The usual cause is either a small, high-riding patella (patella alta), or valgus knees which lay the line of pull of the quadriceps open to drawing the patella laterally over the femoral condyle. Definitive surgical treatment may be required, but on the field it is nearly always possible to flip the patella back into place.

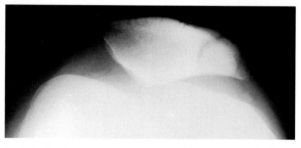

**Fig.126**  Sky-line view of a bi-partite patella in a 20-year-old hockey player.

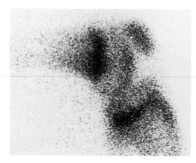

**Fig.127**  Triple-phase technetium 99 bone scan showing a stress fracture of the right patella in a 19-year-old weightlifter.

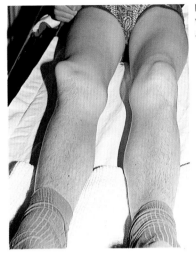

**Fig.128** Right patella which dislocated during a gymnastic lesson.

Pain and swelling in the knee in more senior sportsmen is often accompanied by crepitus on examination, indicating underlying degenerative change. This is due to many years of severe stress on the joint, together with previous injuries, some of which required surgery, for example arthrotomy or menisectomy.

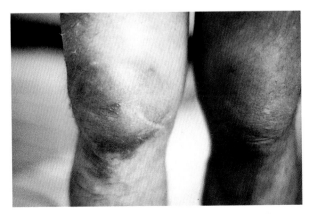

**Fig.129** Scarred, swollen, arthritic knees of a 35-year-old rugby player, who confidently expected to play another few seasons.

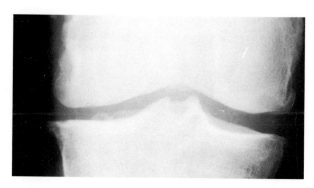

**Fig.130** X-ray of the right knee of 36-year-old football player showing the degenerative changes produced by 20 years of heavy wear and tear induced by playing the game at the highest level.

## THE TIBIA AND FIBULA

The tibia and fibula are surrounded by muscles which are divided into three sections known as the anterior, lateral and posterior compartments. The posterior compartment is subdivided into a deep and superficial layer.

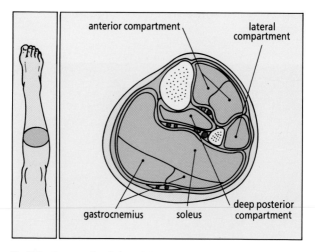

**Fig.131** Cross-sectional view of the lower leg demonstrating the muscle compartments. The muscles are separated by tough, fibrous septa, which are firmly attached to the bones.

The muscles of the anterior and lateral compartments supply the long extensors of the foot and ankle whilst the posterior compartment is formed by the large triceps surae. The fibrous tissue which surrounds all these muscles is firmly attached to the tibia and fibula and there is little room to accommodate any swelling/enlargement within the compartments. If an increase in intracompartmental volume occurs, for example, an intramuscular haematoma secondary to trauma, or swelling of the muscles themselves due to overuse, the athlete will experience pain in the compartment due to relative ischaemia. This hypoxia can also occur chronically where intensive training has produced an increase in muscle bulk in the leg. This pain and swelling is known as a compartment syndrome.

A tear of the gastrocnemius or plantaris is a common cause of calf pain of sudden onset. It is usually occasioned by sudden forced dorsiflexion on an already plantar flexed foot and commonly occurs in racquet sports and basketball.

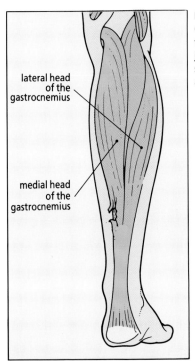

lateral head of the gastrocnemius

medial head of the gastrocnemius

**Fig.132**
Gastrocneumius tear at the musculotendinous junction on the medial side, the most commonly affected site.

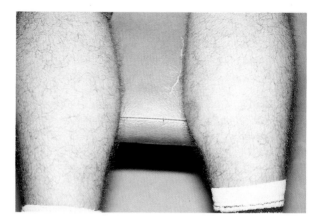

**Fig.133** 27-year-old squash player viewed from the back, who during a match complained of sudden, severe pain in the right calf. Bruising is just beginning to appear at the site of swelling. The injury was treated with support, rest and physiotherapy.

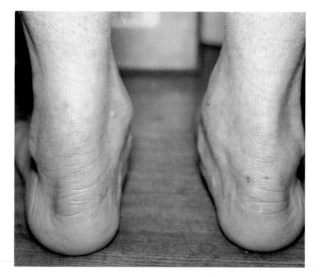

**Fig.134** Tendonitis, or paratendonitis, of the Achilles tendon, which has caused thickening of the left heel of this 45-year-old runner. Initial treatment is with rest, heel raises, physiotherapy and administration of local anti-inflammatory drugs.

Athletes may present with a history of an acute, tearing pain in the heel, which they sometimes ascribe to having been kicked or struck from behind. This is a common presentation where the Achilles tendon has ruptured, and on examination the tendo-Achilles is exquisitely tender and a 'gap' can often be felt a few centimetres above the insertion of the tendon into the calcaneum. The appropriate way to examine the tendo-Achilles is with the patient lying face down, with the feet projecting well over the end of the couch.

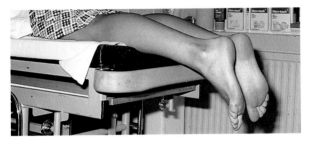

**Fig.135** In this position any defects in the tendon can be palpated and each calf can be gently squeezed. If the tendon is intact, the foot will plantar flex, and if ruptured, no movement occurs (Thompson's test).

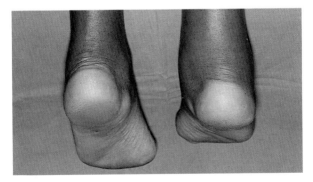

**Fig.136** Heels of a 23-year-old netball player who felt a severe pain in her right tendo-Achilles as she attempted to jump for the ball. The swelling around the right heel is marked. Thompson's test produced no movement of the foot, and an ultrasound scan demonstrated the rupture.

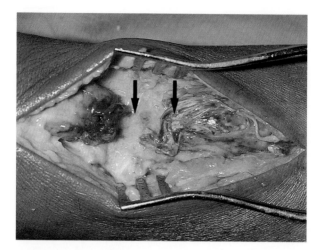

**Fig.137** The right heel of the patient discussed in Fig.136 at operation. The gap between the ends of the ruptured tendon is arrowed. Direct repair was undertaken and the patient returned to competitive sport within six months.

## Bony injuries

Athletes who complain of pain in the lower leg are frequently described as having 'shin splints', a condition which appears to be a variant of the compartment syndrome. However, this type of aching pain in the lower leg, which is related to exercise, can be difficult to distinguish from a stress fracture and it is important to consider this diagnosis and eliminate it with appropriate investigations.

Although stress fractures are considered to be an adult complaint, they can also occur in children who are involved in competitive sport to a high level.

Stress fractures can occur at any site, depending upon the sporting activity and the anatomical make-up of the individual. If the history is strongly suggestive of a stress fracture, and the plain film is normal, a triple-phase technetium 99 bone scan should always be considered.

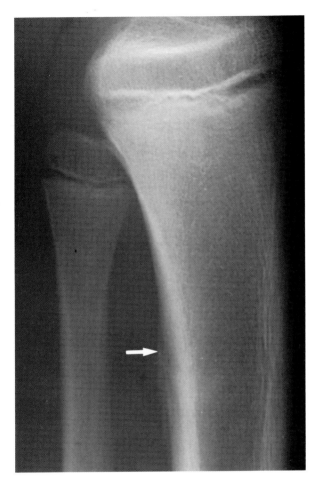

**Fig.138** Lateral X-ray of the knee of a 13-year-old boy who was running half-marathons. A periosteal reaction on the posterior aspect of the upper part of his tibia, due to a stress fracture, can be seen. It is important to make the correct diagnosis from X-rays in such children, who are within the age group which is also at high risk of developing malignant tumours, such as osteosarcomas. Biopsies of stress fractures can be misleading since, as with tumours, they show rapidly dividing cells. If an incorrect diagnosis is made, it can have disastrous consequences.

88

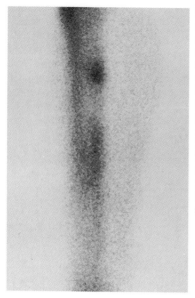

**Fig.139** Isotope scan of a 26-year-old 5,000m runner who complained of pain in the upper part of her shin; this pain came on after running for 2–3 miles. The scan shows an area of increased uptake which represents a stress fracture. The runner was treated with rest, and made a satisfactory recovery, returning to running approximately six months after the scan.

Infrared thermography is also used to diagnose stress fractures. This method demonstrates the increased blood flow which occurs secondary to the area of rapid bone turnover at the fracture site.

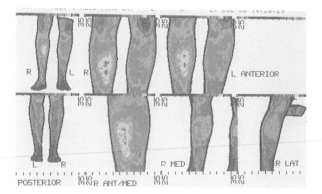

**Fig.140** Thermograms of both legs of a 20-year-old runner with a stress fracture of the shaft of the right tibia.

The tibia and fibula are at risk in all contact sports; however, certain other sports, such as skiing, also have a high incidence of injuries to these bones. There is no doubt, nonetheless, that the marked improvement in boots, bindings and skis in the last decade has markedly lowered the incidence of fractures in the lower part of the leg.

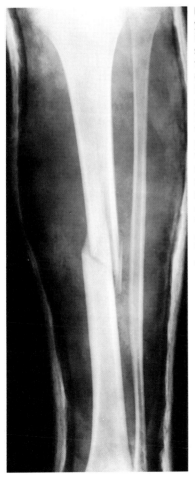

**Fig.141** X-ray of a 20-year-old downhill skier illustrating a spiral, short, oblique boot-top fracture. The fibula classically remains intact in what is frequently a relatively low-velocity injury. The site of the fracture is related to the position of the fixed foot and lower tibia in relation to the top of the boot. Yearly maintenance, inspection of bindings, and proper-fitting boots greatly assist in reducing the incidence of this painful and often debilitating injury.

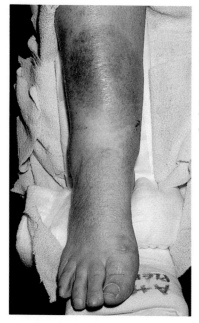

**Fig.142** Lower part of the leg of a 53-year-old downhill skier who sustained a boot-top fracture of the type illustrated in Fig.141. Gross bruising and swelling can be seen, but there is no significant displacement.

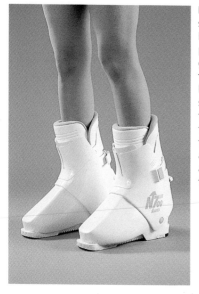

**Fig.143** Skier in modern ski boots. The skin of the boot is made of hard, plastic material which grips the lower part of the limb very firmly. The boot is anchored to the ski. If the skier falls and the boot does not release from this fixed position, a fulcrum will be exerted at the top of the boot and a boot-top type fracture will occur.

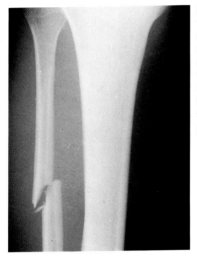

**Fig.144** It is rare for the tibia to be fractured by a direct blow in contact sports; however, a kick on the outer aspect of the calf occasionally results in a fracture to the fibula, as shown in this 23-year-old soccer player.

Occasionally, teenage athletes present with a history of leg pain which is believed to be due to a stress fracture; however, tumours also occur in this age group.

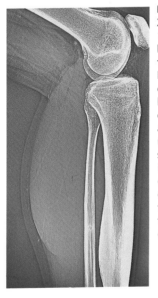

**Fig.145**
Xeroradiograph of the tibia of a 15-year-old rugby player who had experienced pain in his leg for three months. He had initially been treated with rest since a diagnosis of a stress fracture had been made. However, the pain did not improve, kept him awake at night and did not appear to be related to exercise. Marked swelling of the tibia, with an increase in the depth of the cortex, can be seen. The description of the night pain, together with the thickening of the cortex, is in-keeping with a diagnosis of an osteoid osteoma.

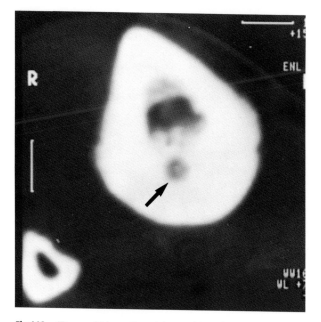

**Fig.146** CT scan which confirmed the suspicion of an osteoid osteoma; this was successfully removed with the use of an isotope probe. The scan shows a second hollow in the shaft of the tibia, which is the site of an osteoid osteoma, the slightly more dense centre representing the so-called 'egg in a nest' appearance of this tumour.

## THE ANKLE

The ankle joint, made up of the tibia and fibula forming a mortice around the talus, is supported by strong, surrounding medial and lateral ligaments. It is the region which is most frequently injured during sporting activity, and acute soft tissue damage around the ankle is common. Injuries may vary from minor strains to complete ligament ruptures, with consequent joint instability. Acute injuries may be seen in most athletic pursuits, for example, in runners and those who engage in contact sports, such as soccer, rugby and American football. Although ligamentous strains are often regarded as trivial, if treated inadequately, serious long-term problems may ensue for the sportsman.

## Soft tissue injuries

Of the three components of the lateral complex, the two which are most commonly damaged are the anterior talofibular ligament and the calcaneofibular ligament. The third

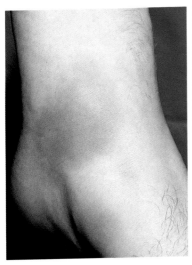

**Fig.147** Right ankle of a 27-year-old badminton player who sustained a severe sprain of the lateral ligaments some 48 hours earlier. This was an inversion injury, and bruising, as a result of ligament damage, is now evident.

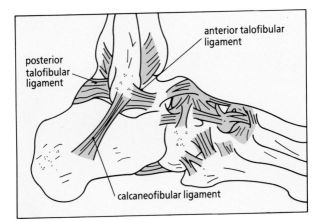

**Fig.148** Diagrammatic representation of the ankle ligaments, illustrating the three components of the lateral complex. The medial side of the joint is supported by the broad, thick, triangular deltoid ligament.

component of the complex, the posterior talofibular ligament, is only involved in approximately 10% of lateral ligament injuries.

Plain X-rays of sprained ankles are generally speaking, unhelpful, even when the ligament has been completely ruptured. However, radiographs are useful when the ligament, instead of tearing in midsubstance, pulls a small piece of bone off the tip of the lateral malleolus. A similar, but less common, avulsion fracture can be seen on the medial site when a bony fragment is pulled off by the deltoid ligament.

If the supporting ankle ligament has been completely ruptured and has not healed properly (commonly due to inadequate treatment), the athlete presents with persistent pain and swelling in the joint, on and after exertion, together with recurrent ankle sprains. Plain films are uninformative and the diagnosis of an unstable joint is best confirmed by undertaking a stress view. The presence of marked haematoma formation, inferior to the lateral malleolus, is a clinical sign which can often indicate a severe ligament injury in this area.

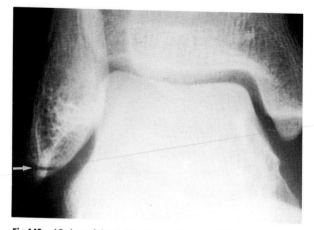

**Fig.149** AP view of the right ankle of a 26-year-old basketball player.

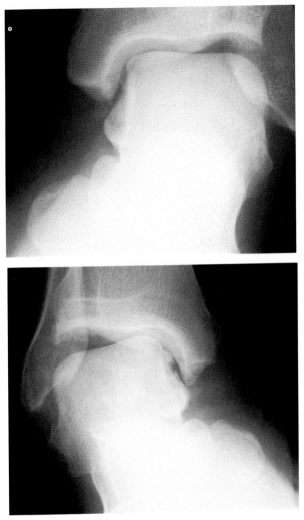

**Fig.150** Stress views of both ankles of a 25-year-old long jumper. To produce these X-rays, the foot has been gripped firmly with one hand and inverted, whilst the tibia and fibula are being held steady by the other hand. Instability is said to exist if the talus tilts more than 7° from the horizontal (bottom) when compared with the normal ankle (top). Intensive rehabilitative physiotherapy would be the first line of treatment, and surgery to reinforce/repair the injured ligament would only be considered if this fails.

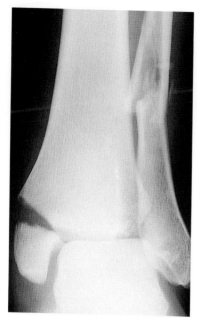

**Fig.151** X-ray of the ankle of a 31-year-old ice-skater who fractured his distal fibula and medial malleolus (a bimalleolar fracture). The ankle joint was unstable and treatment was by internal fixation of both fractures.

## Bony injuries

Any of the three bones which make up the ankle joint may fracture, the most common site being at the lateral malleolus. The treatment of such injuries does not, generally speaking, differ, whether the injuries are sustained during athletic pursuits, or in day-to-day life, although certain sporting activities do carry an increased risk of serious ankle injuries.

Inevitably, if a bone fractures, soft tissues, including blood vessels, will be torn and considerable bleeding with associated swelling will occur.

Of the three bones in the ankle, the talus is least commonly fractured; however, if fractures do occur here they are potentially crippling.

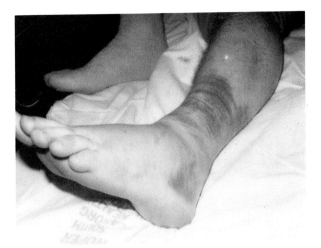

**Fig.152** This demonstrates the amount of bleeding which had occurred secondary to the fracture illustrated in Fig.151; this photograph was taken within three hours of the injury.

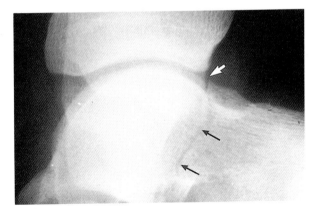

**Fig.153** Lateral view of the left ankle of a 24-year-old rock climber who fell approximately 5m and landed on his feet. There is a lucent line across the neck of the talus indicating a fracture which was unfortunately, not noticed on first examination of the X-ray. This type of injury can result in avascular necrosis of part of the bone, with subsequent gross degenerative changes, a complication which will leave an ankle functionally useless for any sporting activity involving the lower limbs.

In addition to fractures, dislocations and fracture/dislocations commonly occur at the ankle joint and these need careful handling and speedy reduction.

Years of persistent overuse, with frequent minor injuries to the ankle, inevitably result in degenerative changes in the joint, the so-called 'footballer's ankle'.

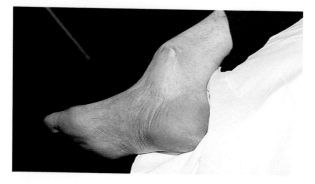

**Fig.154** Dislocated right ankle of a 42-year-old sports master which occurred during a game of soccer. Such dislocations need to be rapidly reduced since there is a possibility of necrosis occurring in the area of skin overlying the projecting bone, in this instance, the skin over the medial malleolus.

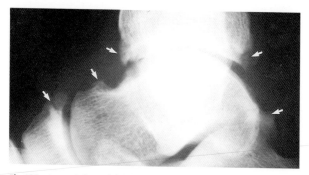

**Fig.155** Lateral view of the right ankle of 32-year-old professional soccer player, showing osteophytes on the anterior and posterior borders of the tibia, bony spurs on the talus impinging on the tibia in dorsiflexion, and a small old fracture of the navicular. All are typical of the degenerative changes found in high-class athletes whose ankles are subjected to repeated stress.

# Other bony lesions

Osteochondritis dissecans, which is found more commonly in the knee joint, also occurs in the ankle, affecting the dome of the talus.

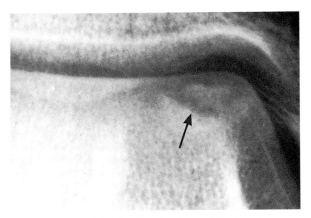

**Fig.156** AP view of the left ankle of a 15-year-old hockey player, demonstrating the osteochondritic lesion on the medial aspect of the dome of the talus. There was a similar area of osteochondritis in the right ankle of this player, whose symptoms included pain and swelling in both joints.

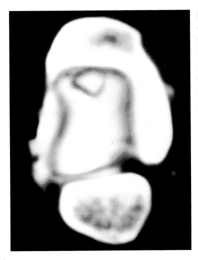

**Fig.157** CT arthrogram of the ankle joint of a young squash player, illustrating an osteochondritic lesion in the talus, the partially detached fragment being clearly outlined.

## THE FOOT

While foot problems are common in runners, they are also frequently seen in sportsmen from other disciplines who undertake a great amount of road work in preparation/ training for their athletic activities, for example, boxing. Both the foot and ankle are prone to overuse damage under circumstances where injuries in other parts of the body cause a change in gait pattern (for example, back problems or hamstring strain). This is also the case where inappropriate footwear is worn, or where roadwork is undertaken on hard, baked, hilly, or uneven surfaces.

### Soft tissue problems

#### Infections
Foot infections are common in sportsmen; both fungi and viruses can attack the feet and are generally picked up when walking over wet surfaces without the protection of foot-wear. Growth of the organisms is facilitated by perspiration, slight degrees of maceration of the skin, or the presence of blisters.

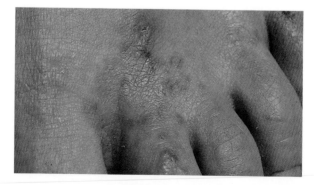

**Fig.158** Typical appearance of athlete's foot which is caused by the fungus *Trichophyton interdigitale* or *Trichophyton rubrum*. This is best treated with a broad-spectrum antifungal, such as econazole, together with strict hygiene measures. Unfortunately, relapse is common.

There are many causes of foot pain but one of the more common in runners is inflammation of the plantar aponeurosis (plantar fasciitis), which occurs secondary to the persistent pounding and stretching to which this structure is subjected.

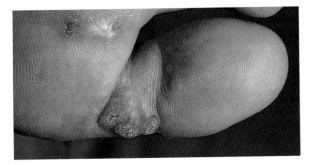

**Fig.159** Plantar wart (verruca) on the sole of a 14-year-old swimmer. The verruca is one of the most common infections seen in young children. Many swimming pool facilities ask children to wear a protective sock (verruca sock) to stop transmission of the infection. The lesion itself is caused by a virus and can disappear spontaneously after a year or so. Cyrotherapy is a useful method of treatment.

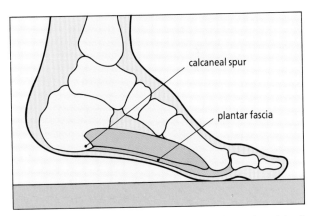

**Fig.160** The site of the plantar fasciitis is usually close to the origin of the aponeurosis from beneath the os calcis. Treatment is by the use of orthotics, together with rest and administration of oral and topical anti-inflammatory drugs.

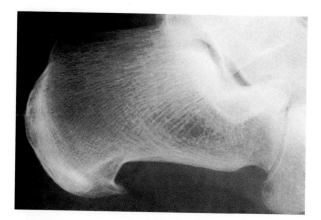

**Fig.161**  Traction of the aponeurosis on its point of origin can produce a calcaneal spur as illustrated in this lateral view of the heel in a 34-year-old 400m runner.

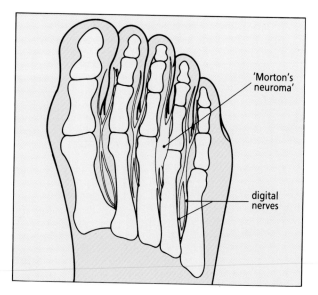

'Morton's neuroma'

digital nerves

**Fig.162**  Morton's neuroma. The common site for these small swellings (neuromata) to appear is between the heads of the metatarsals in the third interspace. Neuromata arise due to repetitive trauma to the nerve.

Another occasional cause of pain in the foot, related to sporting activity, is a neuroma of one of the digital nerves, the so-called 'Morton's neuroma'. This is sometimes seen in runners who complain of pain and numbness in the affected digital cleft following exercise. The pain is sufficient to stop them training, and under these circumstances removal of the neuroma is necessary.

Other individuals, apart from those engaged in the brute or endurance sports, can also experience problems with their feet. Ballet dancers, for instance, subject their feet to immense strains, particularly when they are 'en point'. In this position, they place pressure equivalent to several tonnes onto their great toe, and both hallux valgus and rigidus can result, with serious consequences for the dancers' career.

Fast bowlers also suffer problems with the great toe since they continually traumatize the hallux and its toenail as they abruptly decelerate on their delivery stride; at this point, the great toe is jammed hard into the toecap of the boot and the athletes sustain subungal haematomata and avulsion injuries to the nail, with resulting deformity. This situation is exacerbated by fungal and bacterial infections around the nail.

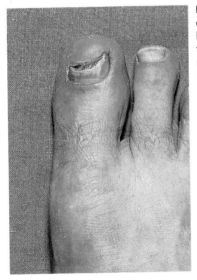

**Fig.163** Right great toe of a 28-year-old fast bowler. The deformity of the nail, secondary to the recurrent minor injuries, is well demonstrated.

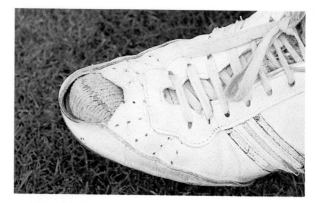

**Fig.164** A 'cure' for the problems discussed in Fig.163. Part of the toecap of the bowler's cricket boot has been cut away.

In sports where the soles of the feet are exposed to shearing stresses, as in squash, small haemorrhages occur in the dermis, the so-called Talon Noir, in addition to blisters.

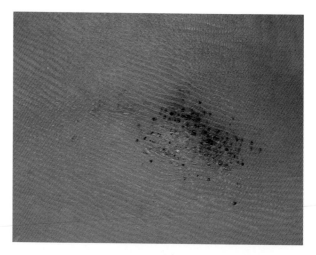

**Fig.165** Talon Noir in the sole of the foot of a 35-year-old squash player. This condition indicates the stresses which are placed upon the foot with deceleration. In itself it does not require treatment.

## Bony injuries

Bony problems may occur acutely, for example, fractures to the base of the fifth metatarsal, or they may be overuse injuries, such as stress fractures to the tarsals or metatarsals. The most frequently occurring acute bony injury in the foot is a fracture of the base of the fifth metatarsal, which occurs when the proximal part of the bone is avulsed by the pull of the peroneus longus tendon when the foot is forcibly inverted.

Overuse injuries to the bones (stress fractures) are common in the feet and usually involve the metatarsals (classically the second), the os calcis, or the navicular, although other tarsal bones can be affected. The athlete commonly presents with pain in the foot, which becomes worse with activity. If the athlete does not rest, the pain becomes constant, being present on walking or even during rest. Often, plain

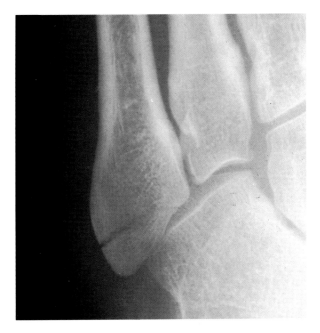

**Fig.166**  Fracture of the base of the fifth metatarsal which has occurred in a 27-year-old tennis player who went over on his ankle on a wet grass court.

X-rays do not show any fracture, or occasionally, the abnormality may be so slight that it is missed on first view and only seen in retrospect. The typical complaint of stress-induced pain, particularly in the athlete who is training hard, should arouse suspicion that a stress fracture is present. In the absence of any change on the routine X-rays, a bone scan should be performed in an attempt to establish a firm diagnosis.

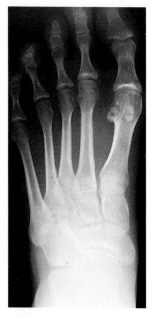

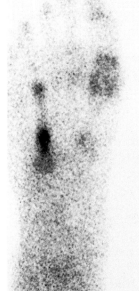

**Fig.167**  X-ray of the left foot of a 19-year-old female long-distance runner who complained of pain. This was passed as normal, but since her history was consistent with a stress fracture, bone scanning was undertaken.

**Fig.168**  Bone scan which confirms the presence of a stress fracture in the shaft of the fourth metatarsal.

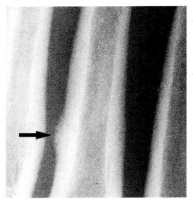

**Fig.169** Close-up of the fourth metatarsal shown in Fig.168, one month later; the fracture site is now marked by callus formation.

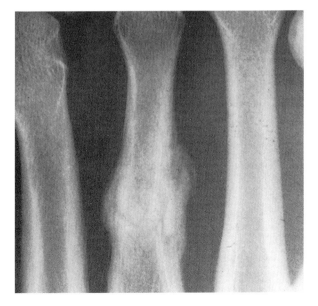

**Fig.170** Typical stress fracture of the third metatarsal of a 24-year-old footballer who had been involved in heavy preseason training on hard, sunbaked grounds.

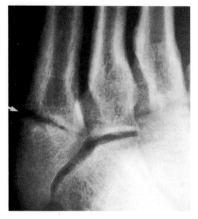

**Fig.171** Stress fracture in the fifth metatarsal, the so-called Jones' fracture, seen in a 25-year-old basketball player. The fracture occurs more distally, beyond the tuberosity, not at the base as shown in Fig.166. Such fractures can sometimes require prolonged immobilization, or even internal fixation since they show a tendency to nonunion.

The navicular bone in the tarsus is particularly prone to stress fractures. This is often seen in females and may be associated with a short first metatarsal.

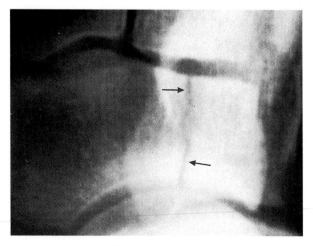

**Fig.172** Tomogram of the navicular of a 20-year-old runner; the fracture to the bone is clearly demonstrated. Adequate treatment is necessary in such cases, otherwise nonunion, which will require surgery, can result.

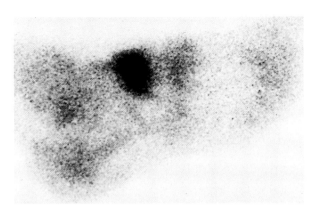

**Fig.173** Fractures of the navicular can easily be missed due to the overlap which occurs between the bones of the tarsus on X-rays. This fracture in an 18-year-old rugby player was only picked up on bone scanning.

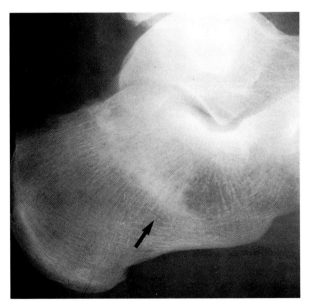

**Fig.174** Classical appearance of a stress fracture of the os calcis in a 29-year-old runner who was complaining of persistent pain in the heel, which appeared after he had increased his daily mileage in preparation for a marathon.

## Other bony lesions

There is a small group of conditions affecting the foot, which are often linked together and which may be found in young athletes. Kohler's disease in young children is an osteochondritis of the navicular which results in the bone becoming sclerotic and compressed. Freiberg's infraction affects the head of the second metatarsal and Sever's disease is a traction apophysitis of the os calcis. These conditions can usually be treated conservatively with rest, support and anti-inflammatories. They rarely require surgical correction.

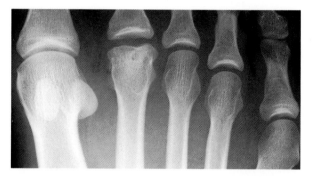

**Fig.175** View of the second metatarsal of the right foot of a 26-year-old dancer showing the characteristic appearance of Freiberg's infraction. This has resulted because of avascular necrosis of the head of the metatarsal, and classically occurs in individuals who place great stress on the ball of the foot and toes.

## THERAPY

Competence in basic first aid is essential for the team physician and physiotherapist. This will ensure that they can cope with immediate measures, such as relieving pain, supporting injuries appropriately, and controlling bleeding.

Some pain relief can be achieved by cooling the injured area and this also has the advantage of minimizing swelling.

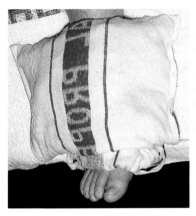

**Fig.176**  Sprained ankle of a 47-year-old golfer which is being cooled with an ice pack. The ice is contained in a thin-walled, sealed waterproof bag, which is wrapped in a towel, thus preventing cold damage to superficial tissues.

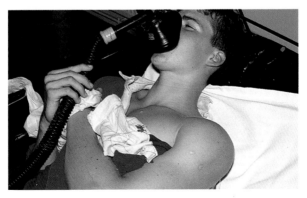

**Fig.177**  Method of delivering analgesia using an entonox apparatus. This technique is used for sportsmen with more serious injuries, for example, fractures and dislocations, especially when the athletes are being moved. In this instance, it is being used by a 16-year-old rugby player with a shoulder injury.

Whilst analgesics of various strengths are commonly required in the acute phase, one group of drugs, the non-steroidal anti-inflammatory drugs (NSAIDs), which has some analgesic activity, has become predominant in the management of sporting injuries. Several different sub-groups of NSAIDS exist, for example, derivatives of proprionic acid, oxicam or those of acetic acid. These drugs work by inhibiting the action of the enzyme, cyclo-oxygenase, thus preventing the formation of prostaglandins, which are mediators of inflammation.

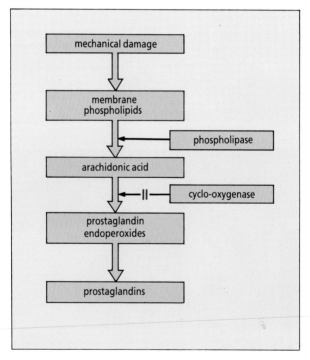

**Fig.178**  NSAIDs act by interfering with the action of cyclo-oxygenase thus preventing the formation of prostaglandin endoperoxides from arachidonic acid.

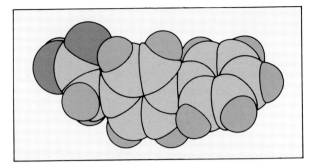

**Fig.179** Computer-generated model of an NSAID molecule (fenbufen). In addition to being anti-inflammatory, NSAIDs also have some analgesic and antipyretic activity.

Early intensive treatment by a skilled chartered physiotherapist who is interested in sports injuries, is important in aiding the return of injured athletes to sporting activities. Various modalities which speed up the healing process are now available for use, including ultrasound, pulsed ultrasound, and interferential therapy.

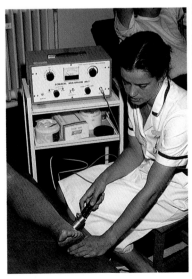

**Fig.180** Ultrasound being applied to the damaged lateral ankle ligaments in a 36-year-old badminton player.

Longer term rehabilitation under the supervision of a physiotherapist/remedial gymnast is vital for those who have sustained more serious injuries, which have perhaps required surgical repair and a reconstruction of ligaments. An appropriately equipped gymnasium and a hydrotherapy pool are essential for such cases.

Another function of the sport's physiotherapist is the application of support strapping to joints, mainly the ankle.

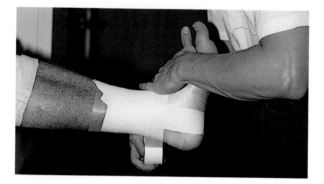

**Fig.181**   Expert taping of an injured ankle in a young football player.

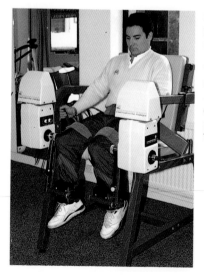

**Fig.182**   Twenty-eight-year-old athlete working on an isokinetic rehabilitation machine. This form of instrumented rehabilitation allows an objective assessment of the sportsman's progress towards full fitness.

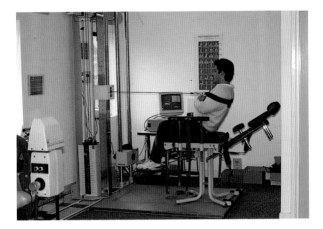

**Fig.183** This static muscle testing station is again useful in assessing the progress of the athlete's rehabilitation.

The use of appropriate footwear is vital for sportsmen who do a lot of running. In general, the best shoe is one which is most comfortable for the individual athlete. An improperly fitting shoe can cause problems ranging from painful blisters and calluses to Achilles tendonitis.

The shoe should have a firm counter to stabilize the heel and to aid in a smooth and quick heel strike, and the roll-off of the heel should be flared and bevelled and should have a wedge component that is both soft and raised to absorb impact at heel strike. These characteristics are essential in the prevention of Achilles tendonitis and plantar fasciitis.

In addition, a well-padded tongue, a well-moulded Achilles pad, and a toe box at least an inch-and-a-half in height, all greatly assist in preventing irritation of the underlying anatomic structures. The sole of the shoe should be flexible in its midportion to prevent calf injuries and should be studded for shock absorption and traction. Finally, the inner lining of the sole should serve as a longitudinal arch support and should also be removable. It is far easier and cheaper to be able to insert an 'off-the-shelf' orthotic than to have to customize a shoe; removability of the sole lining greatly facilitates this process.

# INDEX